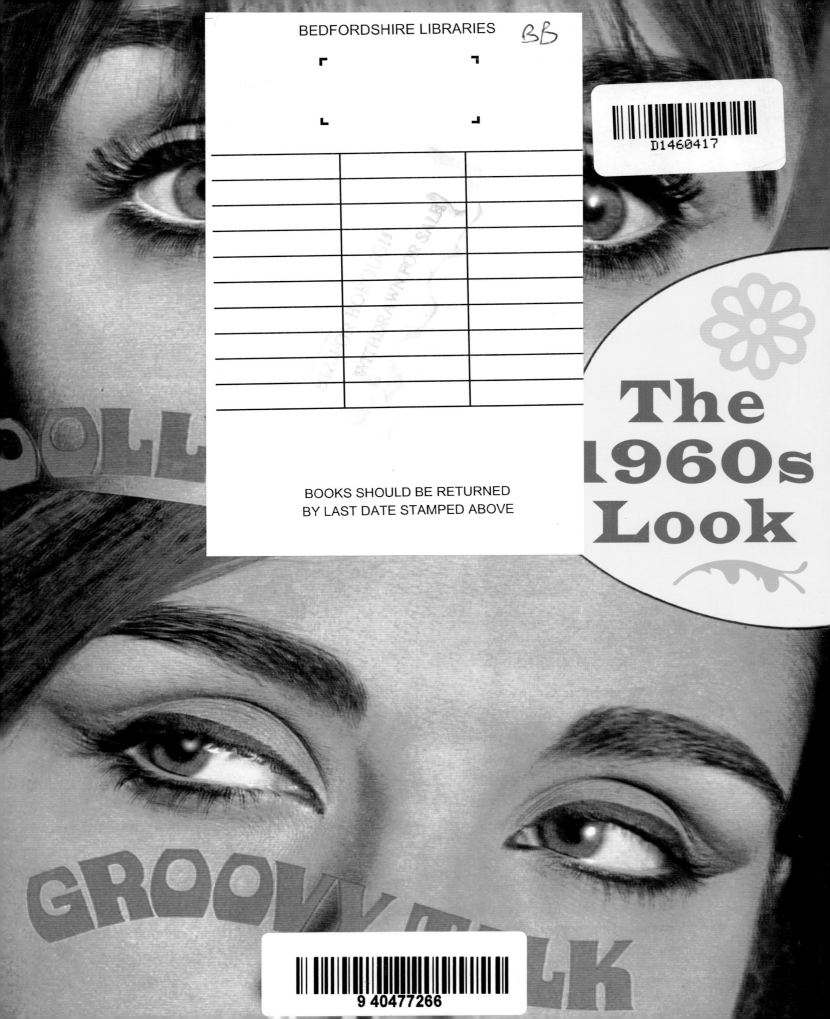

The
1960s
Look

DOLL

GROOVY TALK

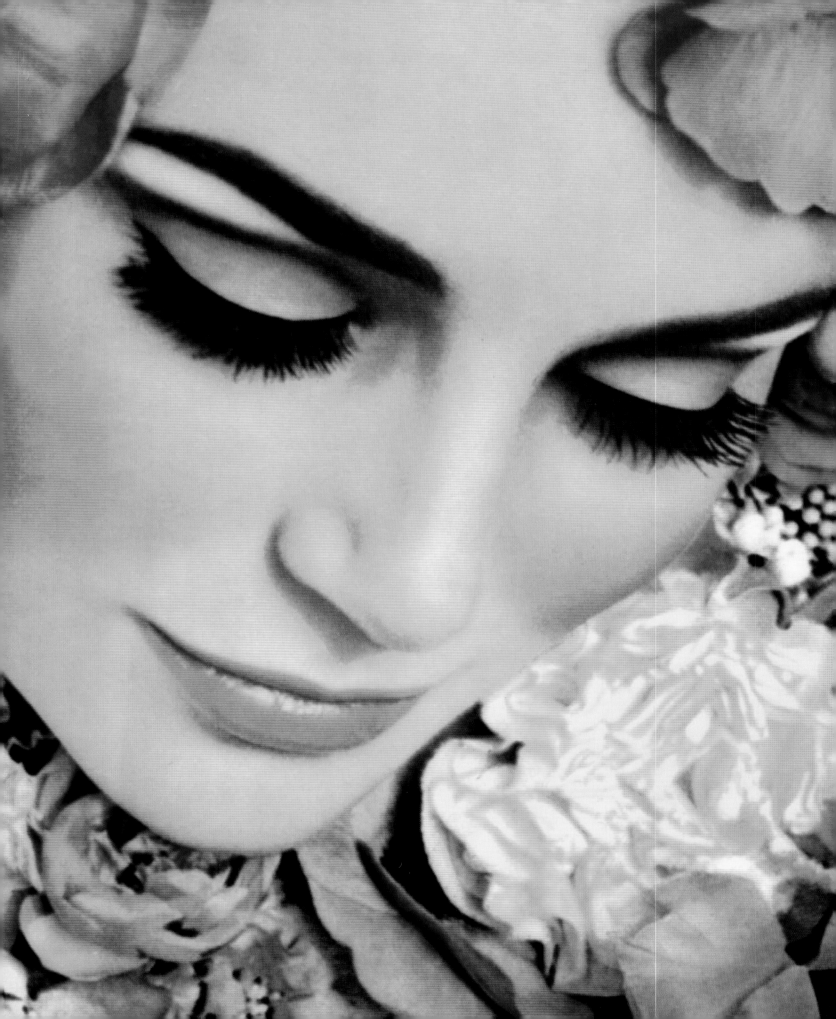

The 1960s Look

Recreating the Fashions of the Sixties

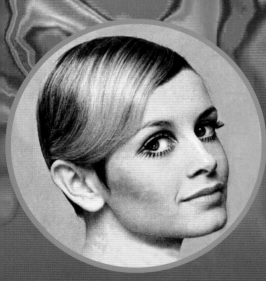
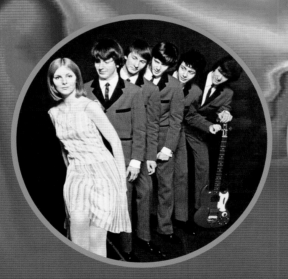
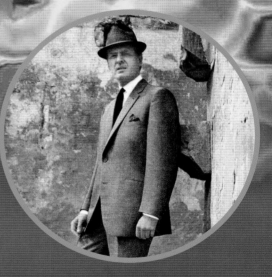

Mike Brown

SABRESTORM

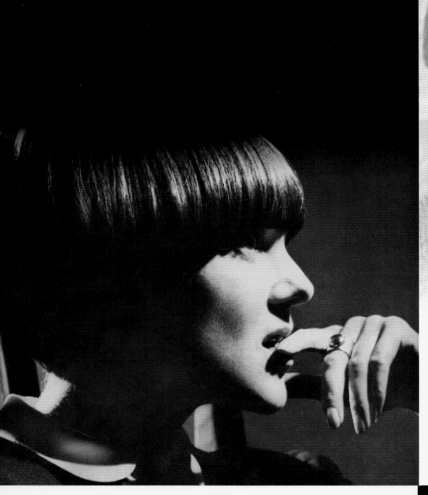
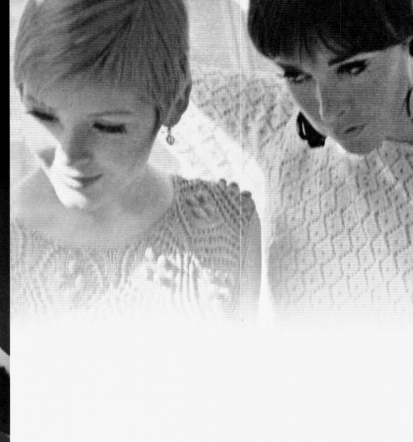

Designed by Philip Clucas MSIAD

Edited by Philip de Ste Croix

British Library Cataloguing in Publication Data

A catalogue record for this book is available from the
British Library

Published by Sabrestorm Publishing,
90 Lennard Road, Dunton Green,
Sevenoaks, Kent TN13 2UX

Website: *www.sabrestorm.com*
Email: *books@sabrestorm.com*

Printed in Malaysia by Tien Wah Press

ISBN 978 1 781220 07 8

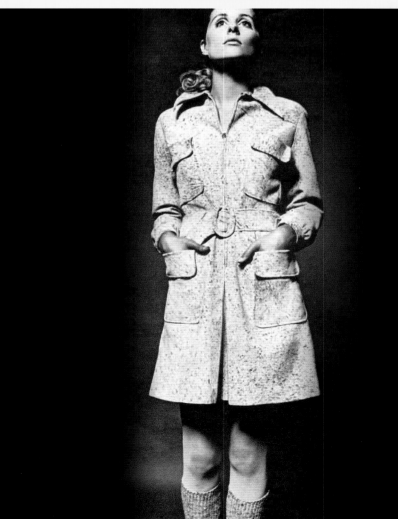

CONTENTS

INTRODUCTION

It is virtually impossible to talk about the 1960s without linking it with the word 'swinging'. The Swinging Sixties, like that other decade routinely linked to an adjective, the Roaring Twenties, was a time of boom following war. In 1957 Prime Minister Harold Macmillan made a speech in which he said *'Let us be frank about it: most of our people have never had it so good'*. Indeed, the 1960s became the most prosperous decade of the twentieth century – two-car families became common, as did foreign holidays and colour television. Fashions were closely followed, especially by the young.

However, the 1960s only began to swing in 1962 when the so-called 'Mersey sound' took off. A new generation of popular musicians, spearheaded by the Beatles, was producing music that would influence the world far beyond Britain. Young designers such as Mary Quant were producing exciting new clothes modelled by the likes of Jean Shrimpton and Twiggy, and innovatively photographed by young photographers who were new to the scene, such as David Bailey, Brian Duffy and Terence Donovan. New clothing styles were created – like the miniskirt – and new materials came to prominence including PVC and Perspex.

Clothes were even sold in new ways: this was the age of the boutique. Young and fashionable men would flock to John

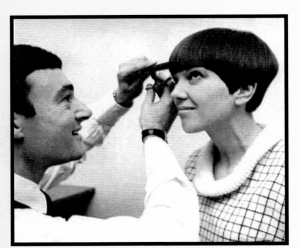

Above *Two icons of the sixties: clothes designer Mary Quant being given the 'five-point cut' by its creator, hairdresser Vidal Sassoon.*

Stephen's His Clothes in London's Carnaby Street; women to Biba, the Kings Road, Chelsea, the Portobello Market or, outside the capital, to the boutiques that opened in every town up and down the country. This was where clothes were casually hung from rails and tried on to the smell of joss sticks and the sound of the latest hits being played at full volume.

Huge social changes took place; youth became almost a religion, with the older generation copying the dress styles of their younger contemporaries. The old class barriers were challenged as a new social order was forged around celebrity photographers, pop stars, actors, models and notable people from all kinds of backgrounds. A public school accent no longer guaranteed success. Indeed, in fashionable circles people with such an accent usually tried very hard to disguise it.

The advent of the oral contraceptive pill in December 1961 – which became popularly known as simply 'the pill' – changed both the lives and the outlook of many women, ushering in the permissive society, jokes about free love, and fuelling the rise of feminism. Meanwhile television coverage of the US civil rights movement and the Vietnam War helped to radicalise many of the younger generation.

Above all else, though, it is through the fashions of the 1960s that the decade is best remembered – fab miniskirts, groovy Beatles' jackets, swinging Edwardian military uniforms, Mods in parkas and Rockers in leathers, plus the hairstyles, jewellery, make-up, and so much else that went to make up 'the 1960s look'.

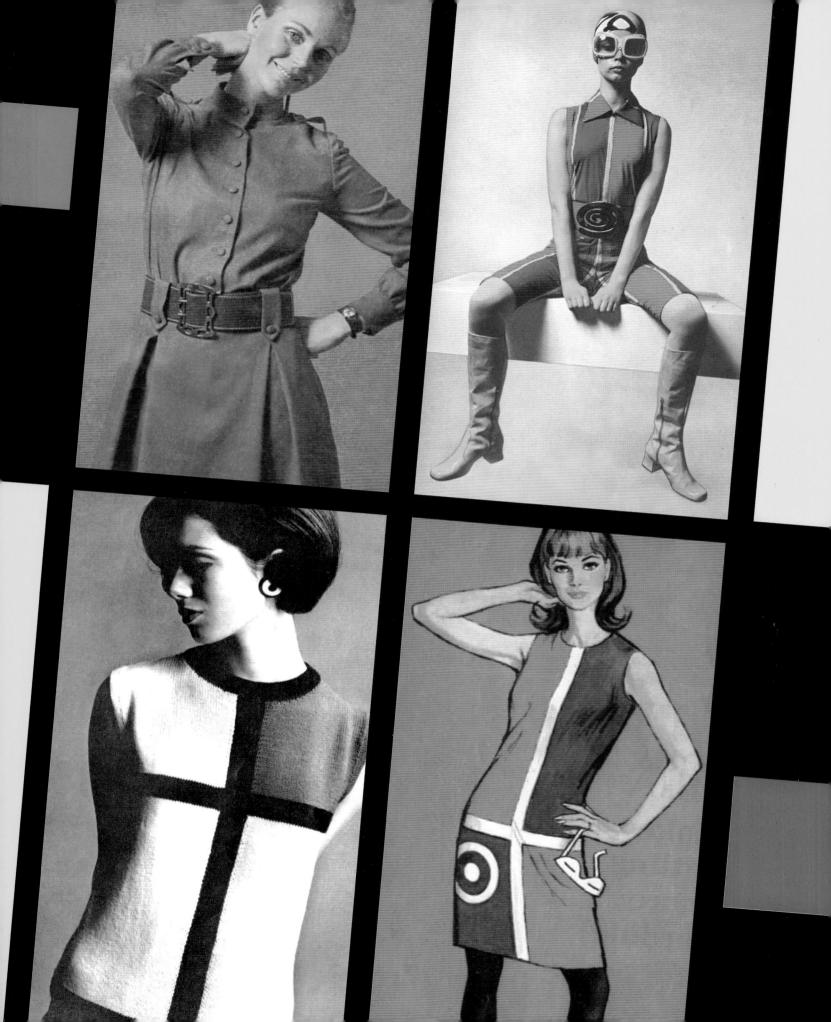

WOMEN

Women's fashions at the turn of the decade in many ways had not changed from those of the 1950s. Tailored suits with gloves and a large, square handbag were still worn on more formal occasions. Dresses with tight bodices and full skirts were common, as were narrow, tapered skirts, but as with hairstyles, make-up and even body shape, the look had softened as the decade came to a close, and more natural, freer lines were taking over. This look was summed up in the 'Chanel suit'. By the start of the 1960s Coco Chanel had re-established her reputation as a designer, and her easy-fitted suits were acclaimed. They were made of wool, often tweed, and featured edgings – usually of

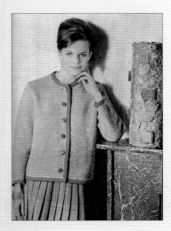

Above Hand-knitted version of the Cardin suit jacket, with typical straight front and bright edge-piping. March 1963.

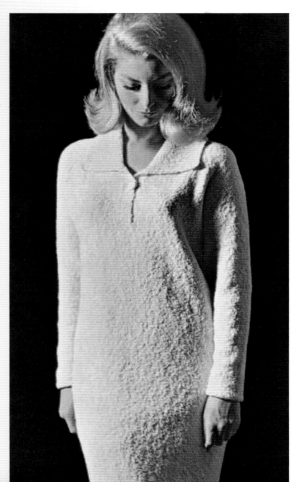

Far right The epitome of the sixties' look; Twiggy, alias fashion model Lesley Hornby in August 1968.

Right That fifties' favourite, the sack dress, saw a revival in the sixties, now rechristened the 'shift'. This one from 1964.

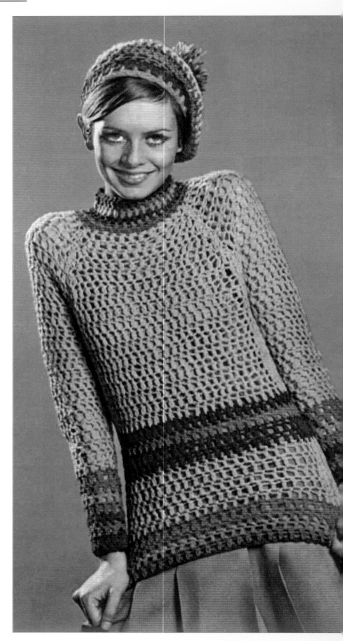

braid – in a contrasting colour. The jackets were worn open and were often cut edge-to-edge to accentuate the look. Normally worn with toned blouses they created a smart yet very feminine look, which suited women of all ages. In consequence the Chanel look was widely copied by the suppliers of high street shops.

The expansion into mainstream culture of the younger style in music and dance was also taking place in fashion, which became younger-looking, freer and brighter – a trend that would continue to flourish and become the hallmark of the decade. Young styles called for young designers who would challenge the accepted orthodoxies.

By 1963 'the 1960s' had well and truly arrived. The rules about what could be worn, when and by whom, what colours and materials were appropriate, and even the differences between men's and women's dress, were discarded. All the existing taboos would be challenged and flouted.

By 1966 this new style of fashion had become established. It was aimed exclusively at the young, and older women frequently complained of being ignored by designers. Styles of the mid-1960s looked best on girls in their teens and early twenties. The fashionable look was to appear as child-like as possible with long legs, a flat chest and a big head with huge eyes, accentuated by dramatic make-up.

Two distinct looks evolved from this new style: the sporty, boyish look – as epitomised by Jean Shrimpton – and the more feminine 'dolly girl' image – as exemplified by Twiggy.

Dolly girls wore clothes that were simple in shape and very young in look. Dresses were extremely short, with armholes cut high to make the torso appear long and skinny, and deeply inset shoulders for an angular silhouette. To add to the juvenile look, dresses were trimmed with frills, lace and embroidered ribbons. They were worn with pale lacy tights and 'skinny rib' pullovers in pastel colours. These were often bought in the children's department of clothing stores so as to be as small and tight as possible.

One popular alternative was an open-knit crocheted top or dress in a soft pastel shade,

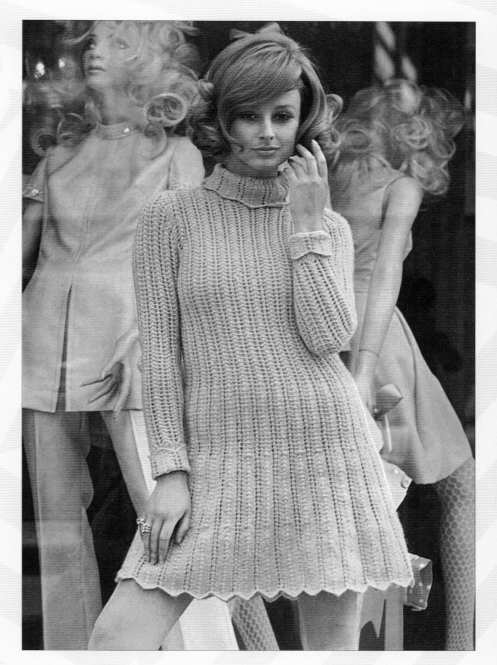

worn by the more daring without a bra or slip. To accentuate the shapeless look belts, often made of chain, were worn round the top of the hips. These might be paired with a small, quilted-leather shoulder bag hung on a narrow chain. The outfit might be finished off with knee-length leather boots, often in black or white, or knee-length socks or novelty stockings to accentuate the legs.

Sporty girls wore boyish styles – jeans, shirts and leather or denim jackets borrowed or pinched from boyfriends or brothers.

Above *The crocheted dress with its teasing, peek-a-boo quality, was a great favourite in the latter sixties, representing the sexual liberation created by the introduction of 'the pill'. This from October 1969.*

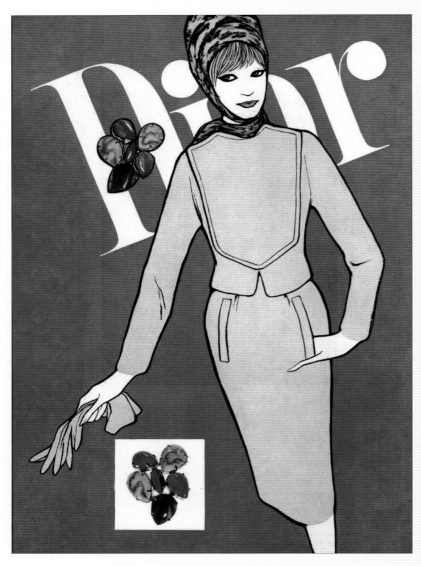

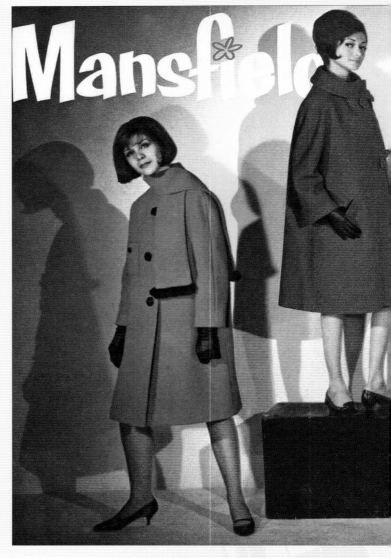

Above left Dior suit from October 1964.

Above right October 1963. Short coats, to go with the new miniskirts, but the most notable thing about this picture is the very new lighting, which evoked the new 'anything goes' mood, and did little to show off the clothes.

Manufacturers soon began to produce men's clothing styles cut for women, which in turn led to the 'unisex' style where couples wore matching outfits.

Fashion photography also underwent a revolution in the 1960s as photographers became more concerned with creating a young swinging image than relying on old, stiff poses which showed off the cut and line of clothes. Models were photographed with hand-held cameras and pictured running, jumping and dancing, with heavily coloured lighting adding to the look. A new style of photography demanded a new wave of photographers – enter David Bailey, Terence Donovan, Brian Duffy, Ronald Traeger and Peter Knapp. When older women

complained that this new style failed to show how the dress looked, Bailey dismissed the idea: 'Well, a frock's a frock, isn't it?'.

In the search for a personal look some of the more adventurous spirits discovered that jumble sales were a rich source for materials and clothes. Velvet and brocade curtains lent themselves to home dressmaking, while Edwardian, 1920s, '30s and '40s clothes were both stylish and cheap. Thus the fashion for wearing period clothes began, although at this time it was done in an eclectic, mix-and-match way – an Edwardian coat worn with a flapper dress, and so on. Some styles, like faux-military jackets, became widespread, and were perfectly illustrated on The Beatles' **Sergeant Pepper** album cover. The feather boa and the fox-fur stole and cape had their moments too, as did the cloche hat. Shops selling period clothes sprang up and from these developed a new style – newly made clothes fashioned in the faded greys and purples of period clothes and made of 1930s fabrics such as crêpe and jersey.

Biba was the most successful example of the new style. It was the brainchild of Barbara Hulanicki who, with her husband Stephen Fitz-Simon, started Biba's Postal Boutique which was run from their flat. Its huge success led to their first shop, established in a former chemist's in London's Kensington. They retained the faded character of the shop with navy blue paint, old bronze lamps and an antique wardrobe. The shop and the clothes created the look, but what made Biba a success was that the average working girl could dress in the latest 'gear' for around 10 per cent of her earnings. As with other 'in' places, its popularity grew by word of mouth – at first the shop did not even have a sign over the door, but there was always a steady stream of customers drawn by the look, or by the chance to rub shoulders with the celebrities often to be found there.

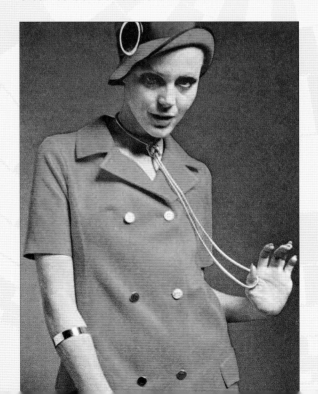

In 1965 Biba moved to Kensington High Street. Once again the decor identified the shop, with specially printed deep red wallpaper, old coat stands, potted palms, ostrich feathers and original mahogany shelves and counters. The Sunday Times called it 'the most beautiful store in the world'.

One of the biggest social influences during this period was the so-called 'sexual revolution'. In July 1961 an oral contraceptive pill was first prescribed in the USA. In Britain in December it was announced that the pill, as it had come to be known, could be prescribed on the NHS to married women. Over the decade its use boomed – in 1962, 50,000 women were 'on the pill' and by the end of the decade this number had risen to one million.

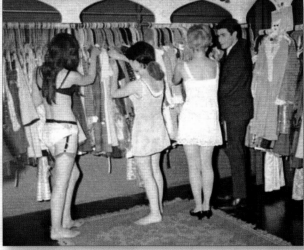

Women were now in control of their personal lives in a way that was almost unimaginable to their mothers. They could pursue a career and have a sexual relationship outside marriage, a situation previously only dreamed of by all but a privileged few (women in many jobs, such as teaching, had to resign when they married).

This freedom was both encouraged by, and at the same time served to fuel, the rise of feminism. Many women now wanted to take control their own lives, which meant they were no longer content to be told what to wear by a handful of designers. The stranglehold on fashion exerted by the couture houses declined sharply. At the same time sex became more overt and clothes more provocative in the guise of the miniskirt, the see-through top and even the topless dress.

Below *Shopping in 'Lady Jane' in Carnaby Street, February 1968. Whilst this type of clothes shop, with rails of clothes, has become the norm, it was quite revolutionary then. Although posed here, it was not uncommon in the more fashionable, busy shops, to see girls trying on the clothes in the open.*

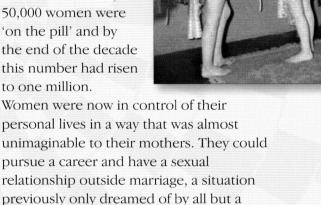

Left *Often fashion designers looked back for inspiration, Edwardian styles were the rage in the middle sixties, while after 'Bonnie and Clyde' the thirties look took over in the later part of the decade. This from January 1969.*

1960

The year 1960 was the springboard when designers led fashion off in many different directions and there was no unified theme. This, in itself, encapsulated the style that would predominate in the new decade, and many of the looks that appeared would themselves set the tone for the 1960s.

Yves Saint Laurent at Dior introduced what he called his – 'Beat Look', which tapped into the street fashions of the young, but used expensive materials like mink and crocodile skin. Like fashion designer Kiki Byrne he featured black leather suits and coats. But the look was not an immediate success. Many said it was too young. Patrick de Barentzen also featured leather, but in his case it was extremely supple and brightly coloured – again integral elements of the 1960s look. Cardin and Castillo featured another look that was to become an important part of the 1960s – one that harked back to the 1920s. It featured slim coats with fur collars worn with cloche hats, headbands and long strings of beads.

Skirt lengths and styles varied enormously, from evening sheaths to a revival of the puff-ball dress, this time shortened to form a kind of bubble at thigh-level. De Barentzen had very full skirts above the knee, while Mary Quant featured what would become one the icons of the decade: the simple sleeveless pinafore dress created a very youthful look, with the added advantage that it could be worn either as day or evening wear.

The March 1960 issue of **Men Only** magazine gave advice about buying and looking after a fur coat: '*Although thousands can be spent on a fur coat, a reasonably good one can be bought from between £75 to £100. When buying a fur, make sure that the hair has a shine; it should be glossy and the pelt should be supple – soft and pliable. With a curly fur, the hair should never feel frizzy.*

'*Only buy a second-hand fur coat from a reputable dealer who is well established –and always make sure you get a receipt. During the summer, furs should, ideally, be placed in cold storage. They should not be left in the wardrobe close to other clothes but allowed room to "breathe". Furs should never be dried in front of a fire; rain does not harm a fur and, in fact, can aid its quality.*

'*Furs should also be regularly cleaned, and when they are not used they should be taken outside and shaken quite vigorously. Do not expose furs to excessive sunlight.*'

Opposite page A tall 1950's hairstyle, but with a teenage inspired casual look of turtle neck sweater and tight slacks... welcome to the birth of the sixties!

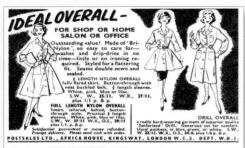

Above The Nylon overall was a practical and up-to-the-minute alternative to the old pinafore for wear around the house.

Right January 1960 – The look at the start of the decade. Very fifties, but a softer more natural version.

Far right The flared skirt, the gloves, the make up, the pointed-toe stilettos, all could be fifties, but once again, the hair gives away that this is 1960.

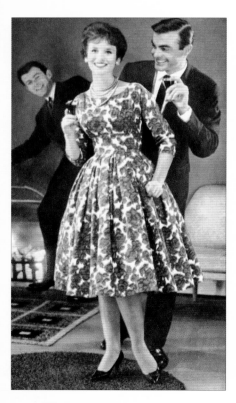

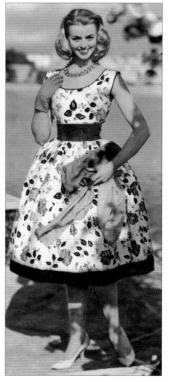

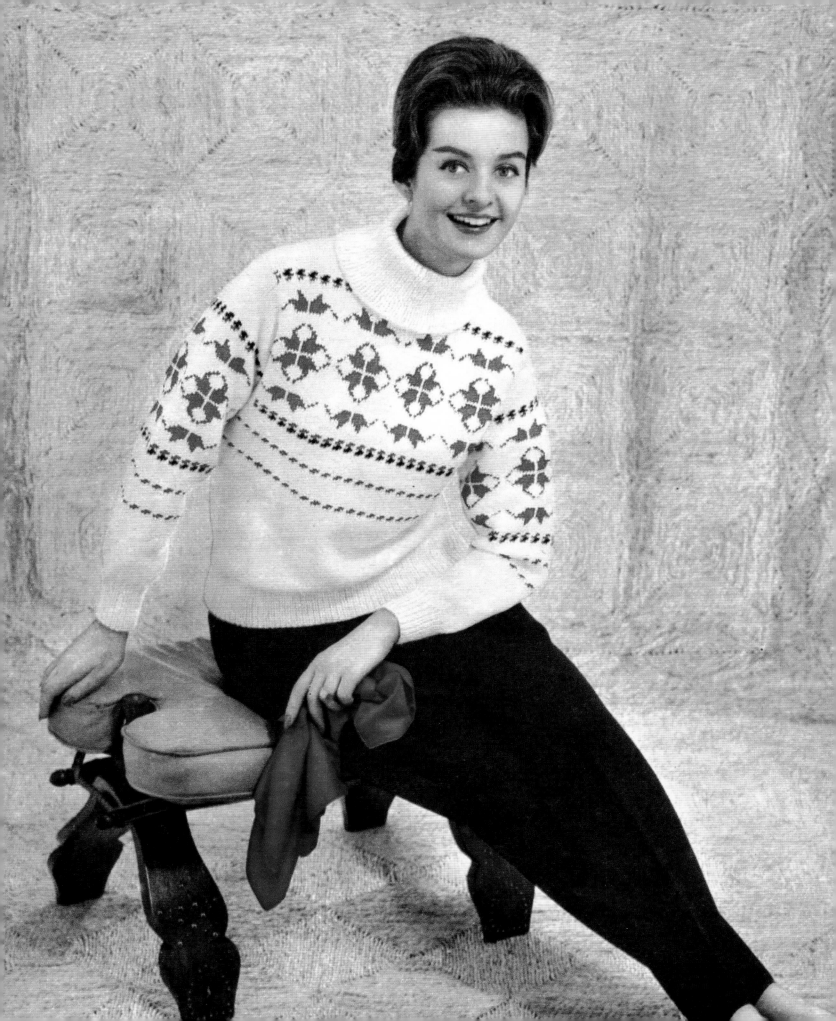

1961

Bright colours were evident again in the Paris spring collections, including those of Cardin, Patou, Balmain and Marc Bohan who had taken over from Saint Laurent as chief designer at Dior. Chiffon was widely used

Hemlines continued to rise, following the previous year's above-the-knee move by de Barentzen and others. Bohan and Courrèges were the first couturiers to include miniskirts, but once again they came in a wide variety of lengths.

Fur was 1961's seasonal trimming of choice, with long fur scarves, jabots and a wide range of headwear, especially turbans and hoods, including one by Dior based on an aviator's cap. For one of his coats, Balmain used squares of astrakhan fur appliqué on a black and white tweed material.

In October Ginette Spanier, directrice of the House of Balmain in Paris, described that season's fashions for **Housewife** magazine. *'For a long time we've had full skirts or sheaths, wide coats or tight-fitting coats, but not for years have we had that marvellously becoming compromise – the flared skirt. And it has come back to us in every kind of garment: from the little dress through the*

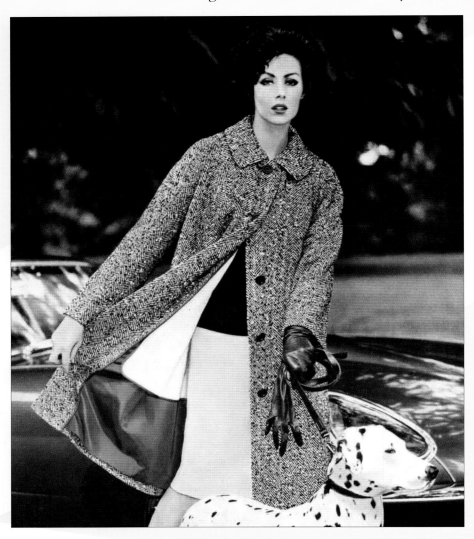

Above *Tweed overcoat from October 1961.*

Right *Fashions from spring 1961.*

and prints predominated. The Italian collections, too, concentrated on bright colours. Bold textile designs were growing in popularity, owing much to the Scandinavian designer Marimekko.

These styles and materials also predominated in the ready-to-wear market, both in Europe and America, with the addition of stretch fabrics like jersey and terry towelling.

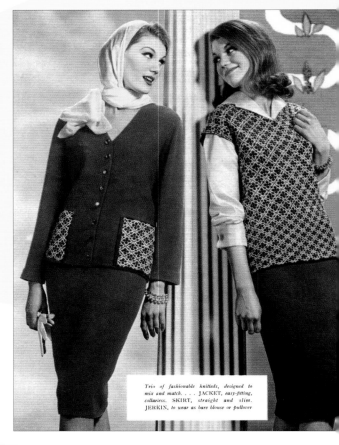

Trio of fashionable knitteds, designed to mix and match. . . . JACKET, easy-fitting, collarless. SKIRT, straight and slim. JERKIN, to wear as bare blouse or pullover

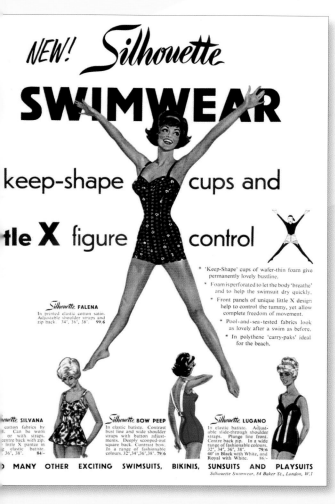

There is nothing worse than an ill-fitting suit. Spend money on a suit, or if you haven't the money, buy a dress. You can't bluff with a suit.'

On the subject of trousers, she advised that: *'You must be just as careful choosing your slacks as choosing your suit. Get well-fitting slacks that do not crumple halfway up your legs, and as far as I am concerned never, never have slacks in patterned materials. If you are not really thin, choose dark colours. Wear the top part of your outfit, sweater, shirt or blouse, outside and long. Don't let's have the skimpy effect.'*

The sack dress, renamed the 'shift', was revived in a slightly more shaped style than the original. Sleeveless and knee-length, it was perfect for evening wear as the 'Twist' became the dance craze, and stylish women in expensive nightclubs took to the dance floor to gyrate with their dinner-suited escorts.

long formal evening dress, right down (or up) to your winter coat.

'All the Collections have bugle bead embroidery on their evening dresses. There is even one House which has a soft embroidered jumper over a chiffon skirt and the jumper is decorated all over with a plaid pattern entirely made of bugle beads. Plaid is very much to the fore this season in coats. Plaids in every colour, showy, loud, gay; mostly used on the cross.

'The black classic suit has come back again after years of absence. You can wear it to go to the office in the morning, and you can doll it up with rich accessories, for the theatre at night. But when I say "classic", don't think I mean masculine. The little black suit of autumn 1961 could not be more feminine with its soft shoulders and its soft, clinging lines.'

But she warned: *'Be careful when you buy a suit. Spend money on it. Where a cocktail dress can be just "cute" and inexpensive, a suit has to fit properly.*

Far left *June 1961 advert for swimsuits. These were now as figure-controlling as bras and girdles.*

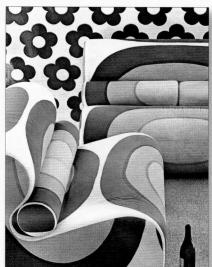

Above *Upholstery design by Marimekko, a Finnish company whose designs were hugely influential in the early sixties.*

Left *Knitted fashions from January 1961. Knitting remained a common way of providing cheap clothing for yourself and your family.*

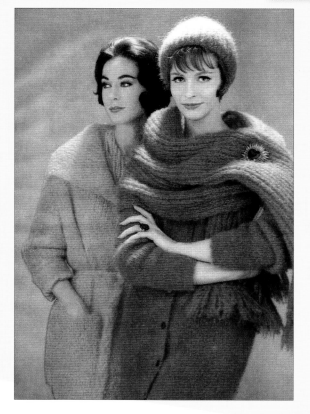

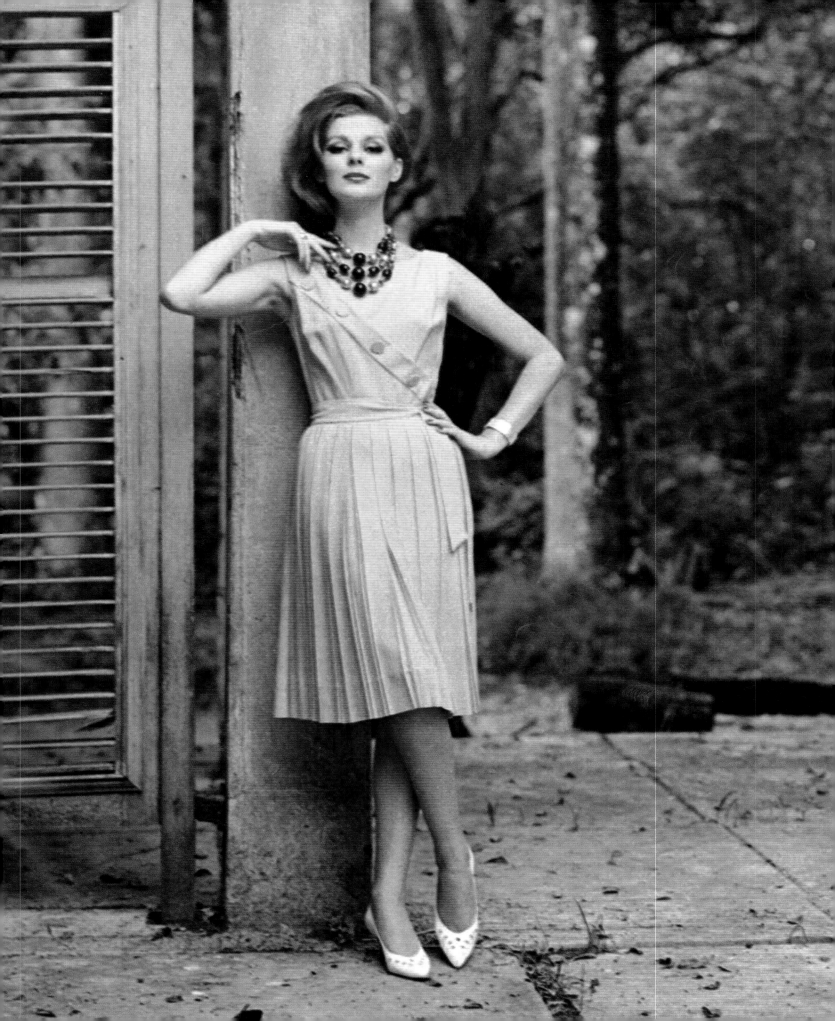

1962

By now Paris was beginning to lose its way. Traditionally the centre of couture, its designers were increasingly following the lead of young British, and even American, designers. Mary Quant was an especial influence.

Modern Woman of September 1962 reported to its readers on the fashions that autumn: *'It's young, it's gay and it's taken wholesale from the dandies of all ages! It's*

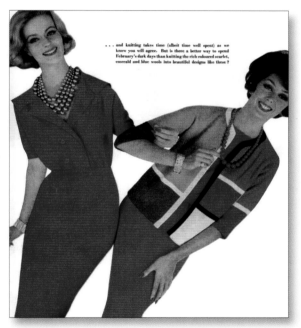

boyish, yet elegant – worn with an air. Chosen wisely, it will suit anyone, for a woman these days can look the age she wants to and no one needs to dress "old". Don't be afraid of this new young look! The dandy influence shows in Beau Brummell ruffles, in military buttons, watches, chains and fobs; in shirt and sweater looks, cape collars and squash-ins.'

After the previous year's bright colours, a reaction was on the cards. Favourite colours for couture daywear were black, grey and brown, and a simple black-and-white check designed by Dormeuil was very popular. There was a return to black leather for coats, suits and even dresses, while Balenciaga's

models wore black patent-leather boots which zipped up the side.

Colour only appeared in evening wear and coats. Saint Laurent's designs included very colourful coats in enormous plaid patterns, and a 'pea jacket', based on the traditional double-breasted coat worn by sailors. He also featured his 'brassière dress', a rather daring cut-out design. He abandoned his 'beat' look, developing instead the gamine style made popular by François Truffaut's film **Jules et Jim**.

A common theme was the return of the waist, emphasised by large, tight belts; it was a look that was particularly favoured in the United States. Another very popular fashion in the US was for unisex casuals that referenced the cowboy look, achieved by denim jeans or corduroys worn with bright men's-style shirts and hats.

Once again fur was in, especially in the form of hats and muffs, for evening wear, boots and an alternative in suede. Even the mini, now firmly established, was produced in fur-tiger by Lanvin-Castillo, panther by Galitzine, while Norman Hartnell produced an ocelot version.

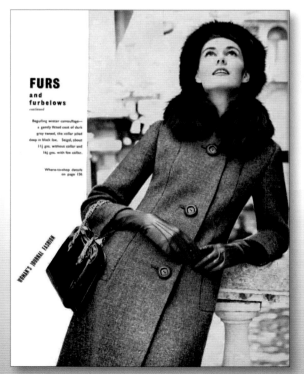

Opposite page *June 1962. The hair is very free, the make-up, especially the lipstick, more subdued, the bust and waistline still on the natural side.*

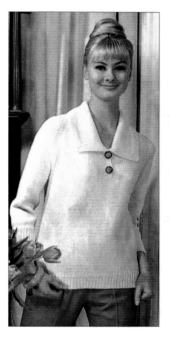

Above *August 1962. The casual look still consists of sweater and slacks, and a high beehive.*

Far left *February 1962. Bright knitted clothes, especially the cardigan on the right which has definite overtones of later op art designs.*

Left *Fur, in the form of coats, trims or hats, was all the fashion that winter.*

1963

Far right *Hats and matching outfits from October 1963.*

Simplicity, in the form of clean lines, was paramount to achieve the young look that had become the goal of most designers. **Woman's Weekly** in October 1963 advised that a *'grey flannel pinafore skirt plus a crisp shirt gives that schoolgirl look, which*

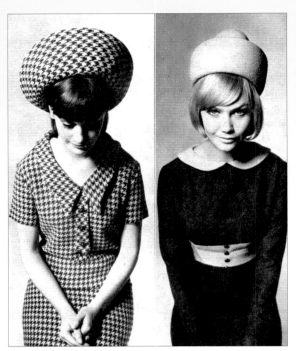

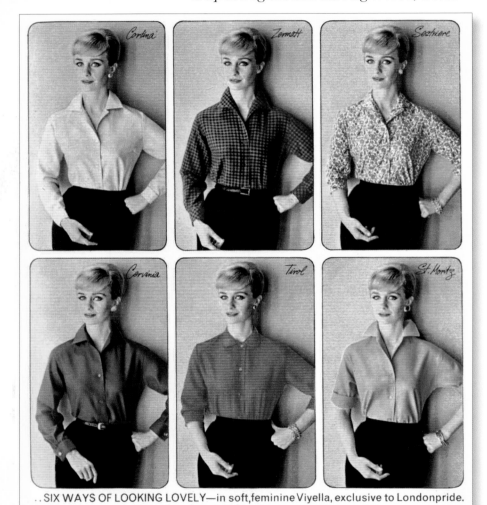

.. SIX WAYS OF LOOKING LOVELY—in soft, feminine Viyella, exclusive to Londonpride.

Above *Six blouses from October 1963, notable however is the make up; the lips, once the centre of attraction in the fifties, are more subdued than before, and the eyes are beginning to take their place as the most important features.*

is suddenly all the rage.' The most fashionable dress was the shift, sometimes with cut-outs at the sides or back, or made with a high waist for summer. There were even leather versions by Samuel Robery. Peasant smocks were also popular, the latter favoured by Saint Laurent, Cardin and Ricci. Other child-like fashions included culottes and pinafores, and Yves Saint Laurent's 1960 'beat look' was revived and adapted.

Emanuelle Khanh introduced a new long petal-shaped collar that would become known as the 'droop'. It became a classic of the 1960s look.

That autumn Mary Quant launched her 'Ginger Group' label – a collection of reasonably cheap separates based on the new college-girl look, which could be worn together in a series of combinations. This meant that the average working girl could build up her wardrobe piece by piece, and that fashion was no longer only available to the better-off customer.

Other looks included Russian styles favoured by Dior and Yves Saint Laurent, which included peasant smocks, long coats with fur hems and hoods, Cossack hats, and boots in suede, fur and leather. Alligator was 'in' – and not just for boots: it could be seen, either mock or the real thing, in the shape of trousers, windbreaker jackets and in fashionably short top coats.

Suits were popular everyday wear, in wool, cardigan or tweed. Checks, including houndstooth, were still in fashion, but tartan was 'all the rage' in Britain. Suits were worn with blouses, polo necks and turtlenecks, boots, matching hats and,

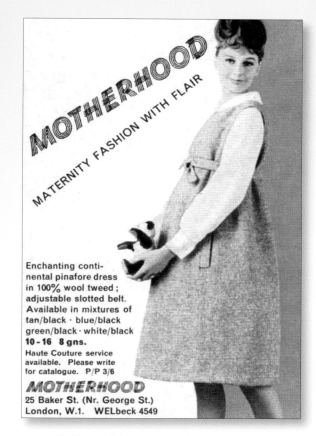

most fashionably, textured stockings. Topcoats remained colourful, often cut smock-style, with tall collars or integral scarves, or short and belted.

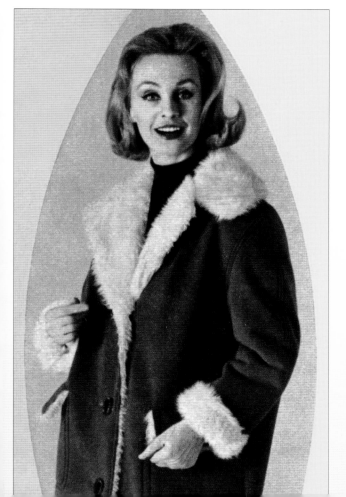

Discussing the latest in swimwear, **Woman** magazine told its readers: *'The new swimsuits have built-up lines, built-in glamour – and lots of man appeal. Petticoat bodices cut shoulder-high give more support or leave scope for a bra underneath. Help give a long, lithe look, too. Little-boy legs, cut straight and not too tight, camouflage thicker thighs. Curvy, cutaway leg lines*

Left Maternity dress from 1963, far more styled and attractive than its predecessors.

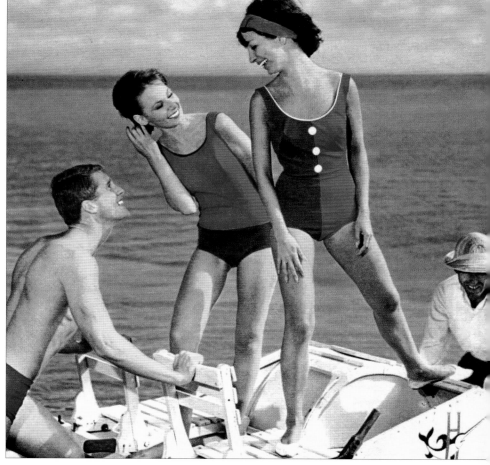

lengthen limbs. Coming colours are plainly patriotic – red, white and blue. New trims are big, bold buttons; buckled belts. Add elegant extras. A jumbo-size beach bag with washable plastic lining for all your bits and bobs. A big-brimmed sunhat – worn model-style over a plain chiffon head scarf. A cover-up towelling tabard. Simply stitch together a pair of gay towels over shoulder line leaving neck and sides open. Tie at the waist with matching cord.'

Above Swimsuits followed the more natural body shape appearing in the early sixties, and the fashion for bright, primary colours.

Left In 1963 the sheepskin coat began to come into its own.

1964

Below One alternative to the problem of the short hemline was to make the pants long, like these pantaloons, which led to the knickerbocker suit. November 1964.

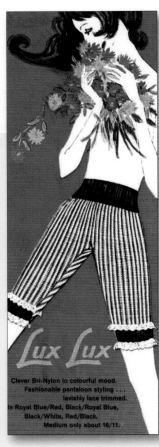

Lux Lux

Clever Bri-Nylon in colourful mood.
Fashionable pantaloon styling . . .
lavishly lace trimmed.
In Royal Blue/Red, Black/Royal Blue,
Black/White, Red/Black.
Medium only about 16/11.

Right Tartans and plaids were often fashionable, as were man-made fibres.

Courrèges' collection hit the headlines. It was a simple, unadorned line, using heavy wool crêpe or a new 'triple gabardine' in white, bright red or strong green. The collection was presented in plain white showrooms by tall, athletic models with very short hair. Most remarkable were a single ciré rectangle worn as a coat and white trousers worn with equally white, flat kidskin boots. Together they had the effect of making the wearer's legs look very long and elegant, teamed with goggles and high-domed flying-style helmets influenced by the equipment worn by astronauts. These and the white and silver colour scheme meant that the collection was soon dubbed 'Space Age'. Many outfits included trousers; those which did not had skirts several inches above the knee, and worn with soft kid boots which, like the clothes, came in white or strong bright colours. Paco Rabanne also worked on the Space Age theme with chain-mail-style dresses made from lightweight plastic paillettes, worn with huge plastic earrings and Perspex rings.

The emphasis of that year's Paris couture was a close-to-the-figure line, with narrow shoulders, high armholes and waistlines and small, rounded collars. All were made with soft and supple materials. Cut-outs in various positions remained popular, mainly on the back, but the American designer Rudi Gernreich took the idea to its natural conclusion with a topless dress, which achieved a great deal of publicity for Gernreich, but very few sales.

Shifts were still in, but with a difference. In March **Modern Woman Magazine** explained: *'To ensure its success for another season, the shift is shaped. Subtle indentations, a marked bust line, the addition of extras at waist level or a contrast at cuffs and collar, give it a lift from the straight and narrow path that it*

took last year. These distinguishing details make each one different so that there is something for everyone. The two-part theme that gives the illusion of a top and skirt is more evident than it has been for a long time. Pinafore styles with varying necklines continue. These dresses are the more grown-up versions of the little-girl look, which is still with us but which many of us are not built for!' Leather and suede were still favoured by younger women who wore them in the form of shifts, tunics, skirts, jackets and trousers.

In the ready-to-wear, everyday world the summer of 1964's **Boyfriend Annual** advised its readers that: *'It's going to be a red, white and blue season! Drab, dark colours – hallmarks of autumn – are giving way to brighter, lighter ones. Now you can colour*

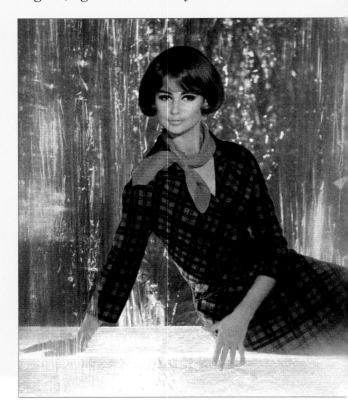

your wardrobe with the rich, deep shades that are going into the shops. Be daring. Buy a red suit with the new longer jacket. Watch the length, though, if you're a shortie. It's wiser for small girls to keep their jackets resting on the hipbone or a fraction above it.

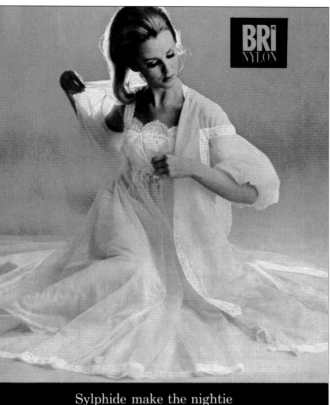

Sylphide make the nightie
BRI-NYLON makes it easy to care for

'Buy a white dress with a long-pointed collar, a shifty shape and a separate belt. Liven it up with a Slim Jim pin worn slantwise on one of the points.

'Buy a pillar-box red coat with the new narrow shoulder line and puffy sleeves at the top. The fitted look is still with us but it's best to get a slightly less-fitted coat for autumn so you can pile sweaters underneath.

'If you are well up on what is "new" you will have noticed that plaids are taking over where tartans – all the rage last season – left off. The Paris-type plaids have certainly never been anywhere near Scotland – those Scottish Earls would have a fit if they could see their Black Watch and Royal Stewarts coming out in red, white and blue rough tweeds.

'As a contrast to the "flag wavers", rich turquoise and burnt orange are second favourites on the autumn colour list.

'To buy something that won't date, your best bet is a pure cashmere shift dress with matching belt from Wallis shops at nine guineas. In a variety of gorgeous colours it can be teamed with the new accessory

shades. Black is still tops for shoes, bags and gloves; but cinnamon, leaf green and deep brown with a grey tinge are catching up fast. Remember, when choosing an outfit for autumn, be different – go for colour in a big way!'

For the autumn of 1964 there was a retro look. **Modern Woman** told its readers that: 'The pages of history have really been turned back this season, and you can find styles reminiscent of Tom Jones, the Victorian era and even the broad-shouldered Thirties. The clothes themselves are simple enough; it's what you wear with them that counts and the fashion tip is to hint at history rather than go all-out for fancy dress. But somehow you must look a demure old-fashioned miss this winter!'

The American designer Rudi Gernreich presented the topless bathing suit styled the 'monokini', and it was promptly banned from many beaches.

Left The long nightie, now in nylon or some other man-made fibre, remained standard nightwear, although as hems rose on skirts, so also with nighties.

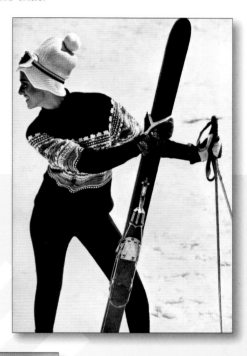

Above Skiing holidays increased. Ski clothing; all-in-one overalls made from elasticated fabrics, coincided wonderfully with the space-age fashions of Balenciaga and Paco Rabane, and influenced everyday fashions.

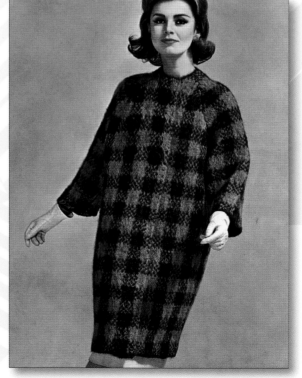

Left Tweed sack-dress style overcoat from 1964.

1965

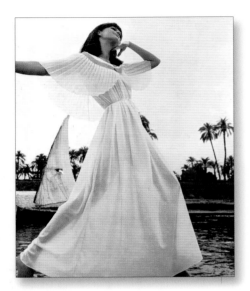

Above *An ancient-Egyptian style nightdress from 1965, perhaps influenced by the Burton/Taylor film of 1963.*

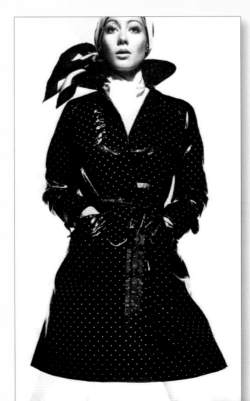

Above *Very much of the period – the tabard, worn with a body stocking.*
Right *Wet look raincoat.*

Mary Quant took Courrèges' 1964 idea of short skirts a stage further, raising them to 6 or 7 inches above the knee. What had not taken off in the haute couture market sold quickly to the young customers of her London boutique 'Bazaar'. Her whole style was about youth; it was neat, clean-cut and made from cotton gabardines and new materials such as PVC. Based in Chelsea's King's Road, the boutique found a ready clientele among the trend-setting art and drama students who lived in the area. Her style soon became known as the 'Chelsea Look'.

In Paris, too, the short dress took off, eclipsing the previous year's trouser suit, while Cardin's new line was dubbed the 'cocoon' in deference to the way it wrapped the body.

Another young British woman helped to shape the Sixties look that year. The Museum of Modern Art in New York staged an exhibition, 'The Responsive Eye', which drew attention to the new Op Art movement. (Op – short for optical – Art created optical illusions and effects using straight lines, geometric shapes, and strong contrast, often black and white.) In particular the exhibition featured the work of British artist Bridget Riley, whose painting 'Current, 1964' was used on the cover of the show's catalogue. She was reportedly furious to discover that the exhibition was pre-empted by dresses printed with copies of her pictures.

Geometric art abounded in fashion design. Ossie Clark had already begun designing for Woollands before he left the Royal College of Art that year. His clothes were printed with black and white Op Art geometric designs influenced by Bridget Riley. The Lanvin-Castillo boutique offered full-length jersey shifts with geometric patterns, while Yves Saint Laurent produced the memorable Mondrian dress based directly on the blocks of colour within straight black lines which made up the painter's most famous works of the inter-war years, such as 'Composition in Red, Blue and Yellow'.

The 'Total Look' was an almost universal theme, with coordinated coats, dresses, skirts, trousers, blouses, boots, hats, jewellery and even hairstyles. The cut-out continued to be a feature of every part of women's attire. In May 1965 **Rave Magazine** commented that: 'Dresses coming *"In" for the summer. No sleeves. Skirts short and slightly flared, geometric patterns. (Circles, diamonds, stripes, checks.) Fave colours: beige or black-and-white. AND holes around the waistband and/or neck and skirt hem. About the size of a small coffee saucer.*

The magazine also recognised that the height of fashion did not suit everyone: *'"In" girls wear good clothes with individual touches. Nor can you discuss clothes without mentioning Courrèges – the space-age French designer. He has some fantastic ideas. BUT – don't go stark, all-the-way mad over Courrèges' ideas. Adapt* them to suit YOU. Don't have your skirt three inches above your knees unless your legs are grade A. Make do with two inches. And don't wear a great big hat if you are about four-foot-eleven!'

The pinafore dress was back, now styled 'the commuter'. It was easy to slip on and versatile; a multitude of blouses or jumpers could be worn underneath. **The Boyfriend Annual** took up the idea: *'And what could be better than an evening out? Just slip off the daytime sweater and pull on a glitter one. Or, better still, wear the commuter as a sleeveless dress and decorate with a brooch. An evening at the cinema calls for something ultra-simple. The high-waisted, little-girl dress is ideal. It won't crease too much, is comfortable and has a really flattering round neckline.'*

The annual also asked: *'Remember when leather used to be strictly for the rich? Nowadays we can all buy the exciting styles that are in the shops, by saving up for the "real thing" or going out straightaway and picking up the fakes. Although black is the kookiest and most practical – especially for cleaning – plenty of other shades are making the scene. Pillar-box red, snowy white, military blue and brown are very popular. There are a fantastic number of styles to choose from. You can buy skirts, tops with V-necks, polo-necks or round necks, capes, dresses, jackets, slacks and even Knickerbockers in leather.*

'A good idea for the freezing weather is to buy a leather dress – with a round neck, no sleeves and an optional belt, and wear it over any light wool dress you have in your wardrobe. An attractive addition to your wardrobe would be a waistcoat in lizard-finished leather to team up with a leather skirt. One of your prize possessions could be a leather skirt at around eight guineas, mock leather slacks at, say, 69/6d, or a jerkin at fifteen guineas.'

There had long been, of course, a rather seamy side to leather, as was reflected in the name 'kinky boots' for the long leather boots that became fashionable later in the decade. The chief drawback with leather was that it was expensive, so to counter this synthetic fabrics were developed which looked like leather (from a distance at least). Many of the cheaper versions had a very plastic, shiny look, but this in turn became fashionable as the 'wet look'.

The Boyfriend Annual told its readers that: *'Although it's great to be able to afford a full length leather coat for around £20, there are fakes at half the price. Pakamac have pulled off a winning double with their plastic raincoats – one mock-croc and the other a glossy city slicker. Belted in the middle, they cost 25s each. They're the latest and the most fashionable – yet they're practical, too.'*

While *'…for one of those rare, sunny days when you're invited out for a drive, it's best to have something gay at the ready. Whether it's a Jaguar or Mini, you'll feel great speeding out in a pair of hipster slacks and a jaunty top which leaves the midriff bare. If you're not daring enough for that, buy a plain shirt to wear with the slacks. Tie a scarf around your head-and you're away!'*

That winter **Women's Journal** told its readers that '…*everywhere there's fashion, feathers are flying – round hemlines, on hoods, even on ears.'*

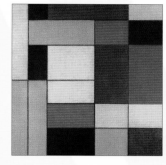

Above Piet Mondrian, Composition in Grey, Red, Yellow and Blue. His use of primary colours was a huge influence on textile design.

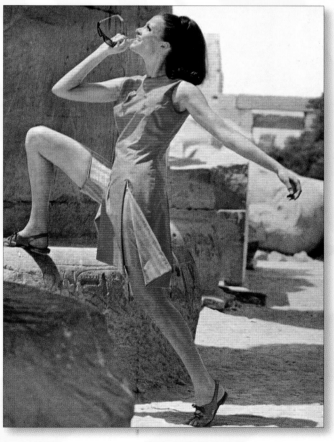

Above Rising hemlines could be the cause of embarrassment for the less brazen. One solution was the use of shorts as a part of the outfit.

1966

Right *Op art mini dress from September 1966.*

Below *Typical shorter nylon nightie with lace trim.*

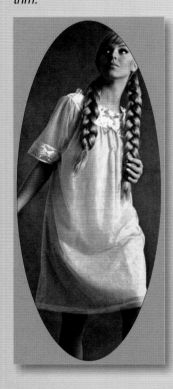

Right *Bikini, left, and cut-away one-piece, right, from May 1966. The cut away started as a kind of best-of-both worlds, for girls whose parents still thought the bikini shocking, or for those who worried that they might lose the top or bottom in a high dive.*

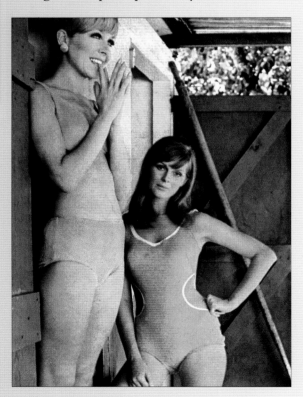

In the battle between the couture houses and street fashion in the form of the boutiques, the boutiques were now winning hands down. Couture smacked of the old, class-ridden social structure where an elite told everyone else how to act, or in this case, to dress. Boutique fashion, on the other hand, was bottom-up and anything goes. In London one of the newest boutiques to open was Barbara Hulanicki's Biba in Kensington High Street.

This new style demanded a new way of looking at fashion, or rather of displaying it. Fashion photography changed, and with it so did the model. Out went the old statuesque beauty and in came Twiggy, **otherwise known as Lesley Hornby, the Daily Mail's** 'Face of the Year'. She was the epitome of the fashionable little-girl look: small, straight-legged, almost straight-bodied, with an elfin face.

Couture did not give in easily, however. Acting on the principle of 'If you can't beat

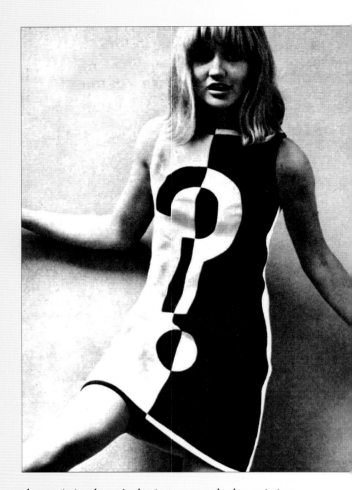

them, join them', designers took the mini to heart, and it dominated the spring collections. Geometry was evident throughout the collections, as was the cut-out. They pushed the limits in other ways in an attempt to regain control of the new trends. New materials were used, like the paper dress, while others made use of tin cans and mirrors. Most famously Paco Rabanne used plastic discs linked with metal rings, rather like medieval armour, to create one of the period's classic dresses. Such new materials demanded new accessories, and in the realm of jewellery precious metals gave way to plastic, Perspex and paper.

In the autumn there was an attempt to replace the mini with the midi. Hemlines plunged to just 16 inches from the ground. It didn't really catch on because most women continued to wear the mini, and most men definitely preferred it. On the other hand, the long coat worn over the

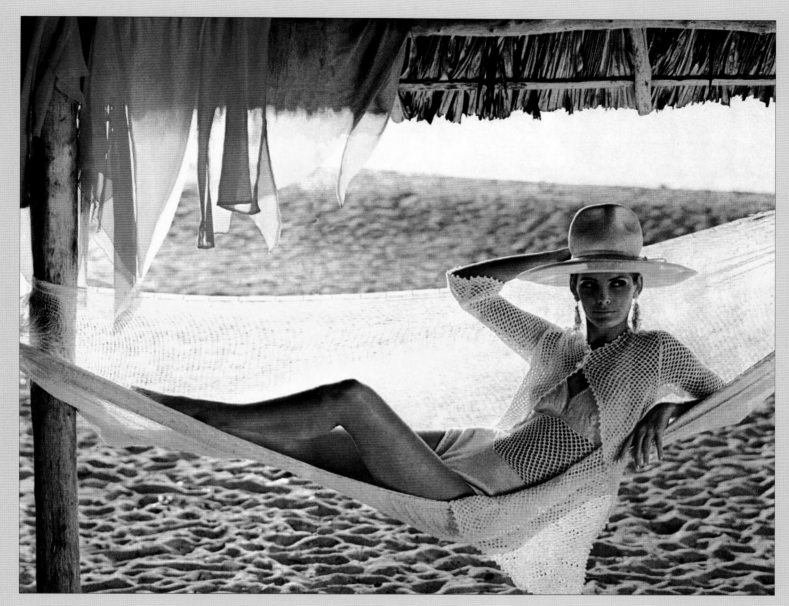

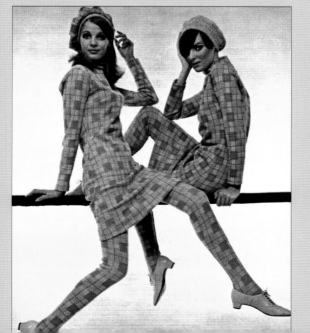

mini worked well, especially when paired with knee-high boots. Again couture tried to introduce long evening dresses, but with little success. Bold floral prints were the height of fashion.

On the streets men had begun to wear Edwardian military-style uniforms, a look that was soon taken up by fashionable young women. John Taylor, editor of the **Tailor and Cutter**, commented: *'Just the old story of women hedging their bets. Wearing the wildly feminine and reaping its advantages, at the same time insisting on equality with the men. They're up to every trick.'*

Above *The crocheted beach top was perfect for hot weather, and led to a fashion for crocheted dresses and even crocheted swimsuits.*

Left *January 1966 – geometric mini-dresses with matching tights. The model on the right is wearing a knitted beret, while the one on the left sports a 'butcher boy' type cap.*

1967

Below A knickerbocker suit. Hemlines were now so high that it was impossible to move without a flash of pants, it made sense therefore to make a feature of them, and the Edwardian theme was perfect. April 1967.

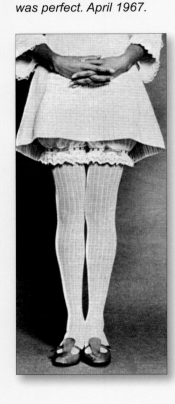

This year marked the end of an era. The mid-1960s scene influenced by futuristic Space Age looks had one last blaze of glory with a craze for all things silver, often in the form of PVC. Jantzen made silver bikinis, worn under floating blue gauze, and Kendal's of Manchester even produced a silver PVC wedding dress. But futurism began to fade and a far more romantic look appeared in several guises. The 'Beau Brummell' style emerged, which was essentially masculine, incorporating berets, finely tailored trousers and suits and waistcoats. The trouser suit made a re-appearance, using tailoring techniques and stiff materials traditionally reserved for men's suits.

There was also a far more feminine style, which harked back to the 1930s, the Victorian era and even earlier, that featured long dresses and coats, velvet and fur. Yves Saint Laurent showed brown velvet pageboy suits worn with high boots, while in a similar vein other designers included tweed or velvet knickerbockers. Fur coats of all sorts were popular, from minks to fun furs in a wide range of colours. Ethnic styles abounded, incorporated either in the form of influences such as American Indian-style beadwork or in genuine imports like Afghan coats that could be bought in the Portobello market or similar places. Shops selling Indian jewellery and fashions, originally set up for immigrants from the subcontinent, now found themselves selling to a far wider clientele.

The Russian look was popular. September's edition of **Woman** magazine advised its readers that: *'Newest lines to look for are pre-revolution Russian – and they're very romantic. Collars are high and small, shape is softly figure-flattering, waists are on view again, skirts are gently swinging. The bell shape with slim front and flaring back is gaining ground and flowing capes*

Right Petula Clark from September 1967 modelling a crocheted dress with large sequins, reminiscent of Paco Rabanne.

are in line with the romantic trends.

'Colours to go for are all the greens from smoky olive and sage to soft or vivid emeralds and darkest fir. Orange is a hot seller from soft toned gold, curry, mustard or burnt orange right through to the traffic stoppers in vivid neon shades. County beiges, camel and brown are back with a dash of plum, damson and magenta.

'Total look to plan for is a fashion must. For the Russian look it means Cossack boots and furry hats in this year's dramatic colour – bitter chocolate. Use the browns with the oranges, too.'

Other commonly seen features included big zips up the front of dresses, and chains appeared everywhere in the form of belts

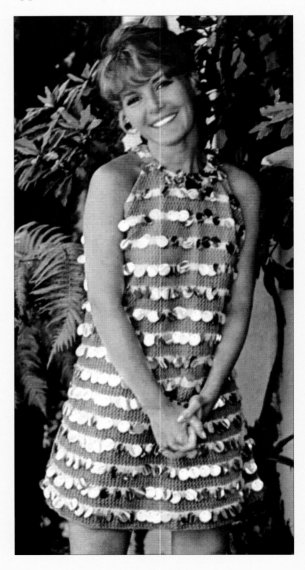

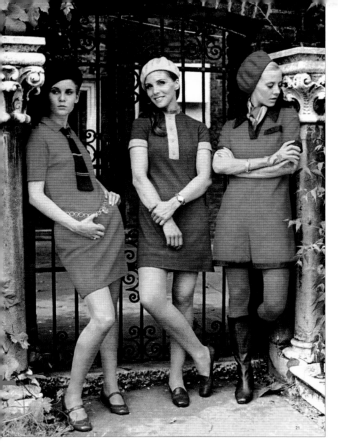

across the hips, necklaces and accessories on shoes or jackets. An alternative look was championed by Courrèges, Paco Rabanne and Ungaro, who persisted with the long-legged, very short-skirted style, dubbed 'bare as you dare'. Bold prints continued to be fashionable, **Titbits** in July declaring: *'Big bold prints have been fashion news for almost a year. The naturalistic flower pattern is giving way to a more abstract style of curvy, swervy patterns.'*

A material for which people had great hopes was paper. **Woman** magazine, in May 1967, wrote: *'Paper clothes are a bit of a lark as yet. But, says Veronica Scott, they will make fashion history. Just off the drawing board, paper fashions are no great threat to the "real" thing. Most are fit only for a few wearings; they tend to tear and split, crumple and crease, sog in the rain (unless plastic-coated). And, as throwaway gear, they still cost too much. After all, you can buy a cotton*

shift for £1 and it will wash and wear for months. But do we want our clothes to last for months? Fashions change at jet speed and everyone wants the newest. Styling must be high, cost low. We are losing our taste for custom-made clothes that date long before they wear out. And paper slots into space-age living. Women expect fewer chores, more leisure; and more clothes for less money, to enjoy it in. Long, striking evening shifts for shillings would mean "yes" to more invitations. Small girls would delight in a new party dress for every party. Mothers would warm to disposable clothes minus zips and buttons. Teens would have a dress for each date. Washing shirts would become ancient history. So far, there is more against the first paper fashions than for them; but all revolutionary inventions have to get going. Whoever liked the first thick nylons? Or the first dull stretch fabrics? Now, however could we do without our soft, sheer stockings? Or the fantastic support we get from stretch bras and girdles?

'The boffins are busy fortifying and beautifying their first paper experiments. Next into print are washable "knitted" clothes. And that's just a beginning. Fabrics have never been more beautiful: we know we would never want to stop using them. But we'd bet a crisp fiver to a sackful of paper shifts, paper will find a place in our wardrobes.'

Vietnam War protests saw the rise of the hippy movement, which began to make its mark on fashion in the form of the flower motif, headbands, bells worn around the neck and brightly coloured psychedelic-patterned clothes.

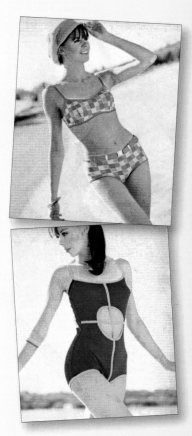

Left *A retro influence in the form of 1930s-style berets worn with very 1967 mini dresses and culottes.*

Both above *Top: bikini in stretch Helanca. Above: one piece with cut-away. The cut-away had now developed into a fashion of its own, used in dresses and other garments. April 1967.*

Left *The paper dress – hailed in the late sixties as the cheap, disposable dress material of the future. This one was by Sylvia Ayton and Zandra Rhodes and cost £1 in May 1967.*

1968

Balenciaga closed his couture house, stating that 'the life that supported the couture is finished. Real couture is a luxury which is just impossible to do any more.' In spite of this the other Paris couture houses produced collections, which were either romantic or functionally classic. Dior featured velvet jackets with tailored, pleated skirts; Saint Laurent showed tailored suits in black wool and tweeds. The classic look that autumn featured Jean Muir dresses in plum-coloured jersey. Coats featured strongly in both styles. **Honey** magazine declared that: *'Fashion's on the side of British weather this winter, what with all the super new macs around. Throw away your headscarf and get one of the new big berets in a bright colour, match it with Wellington boots that Wellington would never have recognised, and fashion-wise you're home and dry!'*

The **Boyfriend Annual** of 1968 predicted that *'It won't be long before we're saying "Gosh, how did we wear knicker-bocker suits?" The trouser-suit is a definite part of our wardrobe now, but the knicker-suits will soon be something we simply laugh about.'*

Both couture and boutique clothes were influenced by hippy style, with all sorts of exotic touches included on clothes, including appliqué that was widely used by, among others, Zandra Rhodes, who applied it to hand-painted felt and silk clothes. Another strong influence was the film **Bonnie and Clyde**, released in 1967, starring Faye Dunaway and Warren Beatty. The 'gangster' look became popular and you could buy designer clothes in the style – among other things Mary Quant produced a Bonnie-style beret. Alternatively you might adapt ready-to-wear items, or ransack granny's wardrobe or hit the second-hand shops.

In January **Honey** magazine told its readers that 1968 would be *'the year of the feminist when women are definitely women. Make this the year you pioneer the look. Boldly leading the field instead of following lamely behind. The 1968 look goes back to the Twenties with Bonnie tweeds and flap-happy Millie Bubbles and bobs into the Thirties with Shirley Temple girlies, and takes a flyer with Amy*

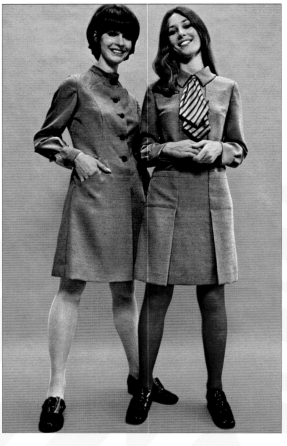

Above *Fashion drawing showing some of the common underwear fashions of 1968, most notable is the move to patterned materials.*

Top right *Hemlines could go no higher and so, like hair, began to be worn longer.*

Right *January 1968 – The previous year's cinema hit 'Bonnie and Clyde' bought with it a new retro look for both men and women – notice the below the knee hemline.*

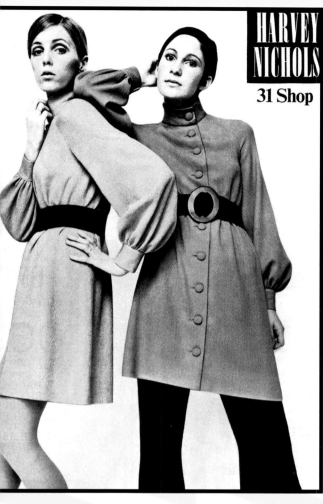

HARVEY NICHOLS

31 Shop

simplicity styling with wild, wild colours. Woollen shifts are another of the classics. They used to be called sheath dresses – the name has changed, but the line will be with us forever.'

Left Jean Muir dresses from autumn 1968 in pure wool, the one on the right turned into a trousers suit by the addition of a crepe woolen trouser.

Below As dress hemlines fell, so did coats, creating a romantic look for 1968.

Johnson and all emancipated women. Go, girl, go! Strike a blow for fashion freedom. Make this the year you checked out in a Bonnie-length suit.' Alternatives included men's-style baggy trousers, the 'droop coat', and variations on the cloche hat.

The 1930s look continued to influence the fashions, and 1968 saw the appearance of the maxi coat, worn with trailing Isadora Duncan-style mufflers. **Men Only** that April advised its readers that; 'Already the girls and the boys are finding novelty in the maxi skirt and the long Sid Field overcoat…The mini is giving way to the maxi only because the mini can get no minnier.'

The **Boyfriend Annual** looked at designs that had lasted: 'Shirt-dresses have been around the fashion scene for at least ten years. I know hemlines have risen, collars become buttoned down, loads of trimmings been added and then removed. And we even did away with collars and went for

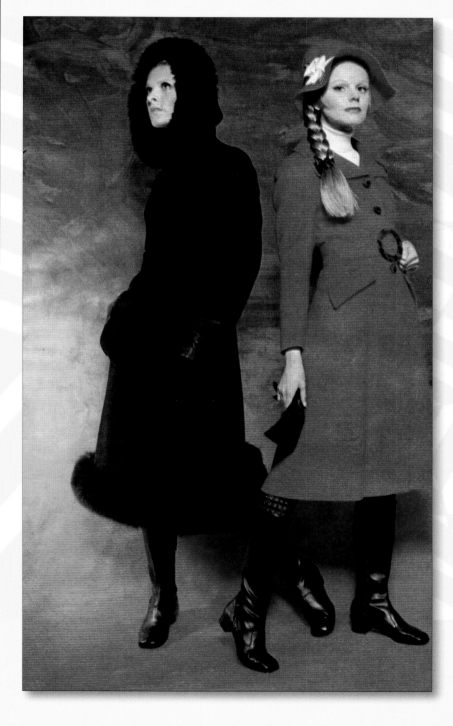

1969

Right Minis existed side-by-side with the midi and maxi - coats as well as skirts. This version, with fur collar, flared skirt and large geometric pattern, is typical. November 1969.

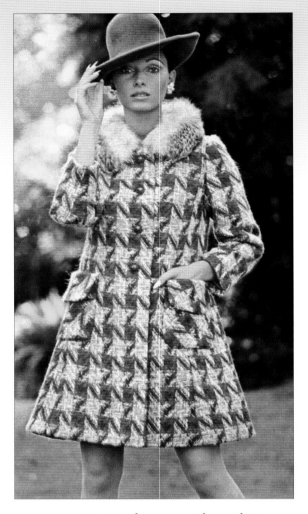

At the beginning of the year Veronica Scott, writing in **Woman** magazine, predicted that: *'Nineteen-sixty-nine will be the year when women will complain least, feel most relaxed, find clothes' care less time-consuming. The message has got home that we need clothes to live in. Not fancy dress, not over-exposed, not aggressively masculine, just clothes designed to enhance a woman's shape and to ease the drudge of being smart.'*

Fashion magazine that January advised its readers that: *'This spring we will be feeling rather fragile. By day as much as by night the dresses we wear will make much of a curvy bosom, a well-defined waist. This spring soft, molten fabrics are swirled up into flippy pleats, controlled by intricate seaming to hug the rib-cage close and used to launch the big beautiful sleeve, seen by day in fluid crêpes and practically weightless wools and by night in a galaxy of diaphanous sheers – silk, chiffon and mousseline, veiling bare arms and deeply cuffed to delineate a slender wrist, and fingers weighed down by a glitter of rings. Coats have cut out their erstwhile military swagger. Fabrics come in all the pearly opalescent pastels of the spring. Vanished without trace are all signs of jazzy razzmatazz. The patterns that dapple all of this spring's delicate floaty fabrics are cloudy swirls of soft pearly colour or prints of Eastern origin both exotic and precise.*

'The look that's universal is waisted, curvy and incorporates pleats. They add kick to coats, provide added emphasis on a waisted daydress and go hand in hand with long curved jackets to reinstate the prettiest look in suits this spring.

'Gone that '68 swagger; back in fashion the guileless simplicity, the good-little girl look, that is neat and shapely and as innocent as peaches and cream. When can

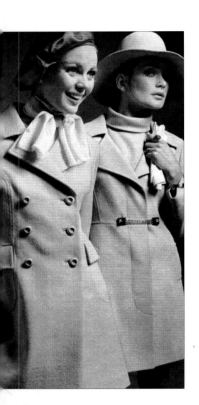

Above A thirties inspired retro look from April 1969.

you wear a pants-dress or rather, when can't you? Well, we wouldn't recommend it at the sort of junket when decorations will be worn but at practically any other time the pants-dress makes beautiful sense.'

Once again show-business created the fashions that year. The musical **Hair** opened, became an instant hit and brought with it American hippy cool, including bead work and Afro hairstyles.

There was no agreement in the couture collections as to the hemline with minis, midis and maxis all on show, and even blends of the mini and maxi: long skirts slit to the thigh, or unbuttoned almost to the top, often worn with shorts underneath. Another variation was a long coat worn over a short dress or skirt. Deep décolletés were another variation on the theme; Cardin's white, pailletted 'Merveilleuse' dress was the most extreme example, cut so low as to reveal all over a rounded directoire neck-line.

Fur, real fur, was hugely fashionable, but as Anne Lambton warned in the **Woman's Journal** in November: *'A fur coat is an asset only if you have plenty of opportunity to wear it. On the other hand, outfits tend to go out of date. I think a good top coat must be first on anyone's list, and next an elegant handbag. After this I would choose a very feminine evening skirt with two super blouses, plus an evening bag. Because I travel a great deal, I have found that my jewel-embroidered caftan is marvellous for parties, but if I were living in the country I would spend the money on*

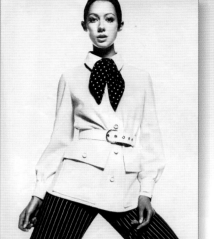

a fleece-lined jacket and boots.'

The 1960s had been a decade of increasingly bottom-up, anti-establishment, anti-couture street fashion, where much of the attention was focused on ordinary working girls and women. Yet this did not mean that the old order had completely disappeared. **Country Life Magazine** told its readers in October about: *'This trend, away from the elaborate and grand towards a much more relaxed and softened look, is particularly obvious this season if one studies the clothes one finds in our top dress salons and boutiques. In these select places, where the county set regularly shop and the jet travellers call in on their flying visits to London, one can find racks of evening clothes that are far from the ornate wonders of yesterday, but still full of quiet elegance and casual opulence.*

'In shops like Tsarina, "O", Simone Mirman and Ian Thomas, all situated within the fashionable boundaries of Chelsea and Knightsbridge, original models at well below couture prices are the big draw. Also, as these places cater for a social life in which the evening plays an important part, evening and cocktail dresses figure most strongly in their collections.'

The magazine looked at 'a youthful evening outfit' designed by Ossie Clark at Quorum which *'illustrates the contemporary evening look on a much cheaper and younger scale. It combines, one might venture to say, hippy sophistication with an originality that is really eye-catching and completely in step with the present mood. Ossie Clark has a great feeling for fluid clothes, and is a leader in this direction among the young London set.'*

Left *Wide trousers and jacket/top from January 1969.*

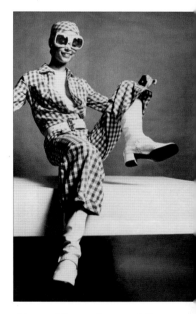

Above *The epitome of the late sixties trouser suit – whacky and fun.*

Left *The fashionable velvets, brocades and silks of the late sixties lent themselves perfectly to formal wear. November 1969.*

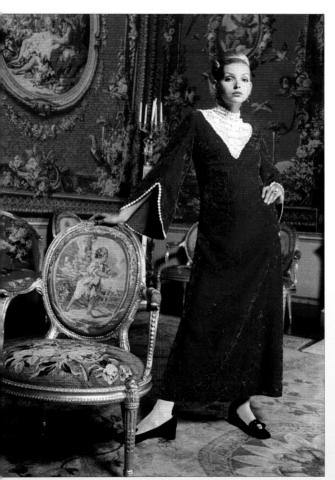

MEN

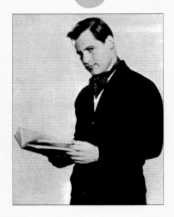

Above Typical men's casual wear from October 1961 – the cardigan was a perennial favourite.

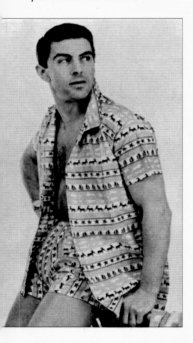

Above Cotton shirt and shorts May 1961, more colourful casual clothing would slowly spread into everyday dress.

In the 1950s it had been teenage boys, rather than girls, whose clothes were so markedly different from their fathers' more conservative look. This trend was continued by teenagers in the 1960s. The popularity of youth culture meant that women below the age of forty sought a younger look, and as the decade progressed so too did their husbands who wore more modern, younger styles. Longer hair, brightly coloured, even patterned shirts, no ties and narrow-cut trousers became commonplace.

Older, more conservative men clung on to the traditions and clothing styles which had remained almost unchanged since the late 1940s, believing that overt sartorial display in the form of coloured shirts, long hair and even aftershave were distinctly effeminate. Yet as the decade wore on, even such bastions of conservatism as the City and the armed forces were to be slowly dragged out of their shells by the 'peacock revolution'.

Homosexuality, while remaining illegal until 1967, was, if not more accepted, at least a little more tolerated as the youthful, more liberal attitudes which would epitomise the 1960s began to emerge. Some braver gay men began to rebel against the old 'keep-your-head-down' attitude, and dressed in more flamboyant styles. Central to this were a few menswear shops in London's Soho such as Bill Green's Vince, which sold shirts in bright colours like yellow, purple and scarlet. Soho was then a melting pot where a strange mixture of gays, gangsters, artists and musicians rubbed shoulders, and shops like Vince catered to a wide clientele, selling shirts, jeans and low-waisted trousers,

known as 'hipsters' or 'hiphuggers'. It was in these shops that pop groups, seeking distinctive stage outfits, found cheap, eye-catching clothes.

It was this link to the music industry that had the biggest effect, as groups influenced youth fashions which in turn affected styles for older men. Famously flamboyant dressers included the Rolling Stones who sported frills, velvet and, for the time, outrageously long hair, and later, Jimi Hendrix, in headband, Afghan coat, velvet trousers and American Indian boots and beadwork.

During the 1960s the long-established men's clothiers Turnbull & Asser became the clothes suppliers to the Swinging London set under the designer Michael Fish, who favoured vibrant colours and modern design. In 1962 they began to supply the outfits for James Bond in the person of Sean Connery, who wore dress shirts with turn-back cuffs fastened with buttons as opposed to cufflinks. They were sometimes referred to as a James Bond cuff. In 1966 Fish opened his own boutique, Mr. Fish, in Piccadilly's Clifford Street, at the bottom of Savile Row. It soon became the place where the 'beautiful people' like David Mlinaric and Lord Lichfield bought their clothes.

Other highly fashionable boutiques included I was Lord Kitchener's Valet in the Portobello Road which specialised in selling second-hand Edwardian-style regimental uniforms. Another 'in' boutique specialising in hippy clothes was Granny Takes a Trip, which opened in Chelsea's Kings Road in February 1966.

Yet cool as the Portobello and King's Roads were, the swinging 1960s scene was summed up by one place – Carnaby Street. In the mid-1950s it had been a down-at-heel area full of cheap tailor's shops. Its rise began in the late 1950s when John Stephen, a Glaswegian ex-welder's apprentice who had worked at Vince, opened a men's boutique called His Clothes at no. 5 Carnaby Street, making up his designs in the back of the premises

It was the Mods who first discovered His Clothes in their search for off-the-peg Italian suits and shoes. Better-off Mods could afford to have their suits and shirts made by tailors, but most of them were not so affluent, so John Stephen stepped in and became know as the 'outfitter to the Mods', catering to both the Mods and their favourite bands, such as the Small Faces.

By 1961 he had four shops in Carnaby Street, four years later this had doubled to eight, and soon it was 15. By 1965 he had expanded outside the area with ten Lord John shops in London and two in Brighton. The press dubbed Stephen the 'King of Carnaby Street' and Mary Quant, said 'He made Carnaby Street. He was Carnaby Street. He invented a look for young men which was wildly exuberant, dashing and fun.'

Stephen introduced a whole new way of selling men's clothes, with garments displayed on rails rather than behind the counter. Customers were encouraged to try them on by young, fashionable sales staff to the sound of the latest hits pounding out at maximum volume. This was a world away from the traditional gentleman's outfitters, and the shops became places to be seen and in which to meet friends.

Stephen did not have a monopoly. Carnaby Street was now the place to shop, and His Clothes was joined by such boutiques

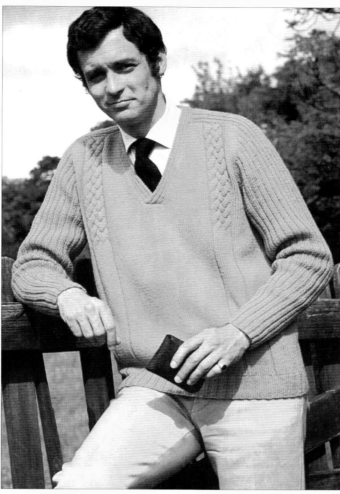

as Topper, the Carnaby Cavern, the Pallisades Boutique and I Was Lord Kitchener's Valet. Up to 1967, the Street catered almost exclusively for men, then Irvine Sellar, owner of Mates, introduced the idea of a single boutique catering to both men and women. It proved another great success. Later Henry Moss and Harry Fox opened a boutique to cater for women opposite Lord John, which they called Lady Jane.

Carnaby Street became, for a while, the centre of Swinging London, but ironically this success sealed its fate. It became more of a tourist attraction than a fashion centre, with more and more of its shops just selling expensive souvenirs.

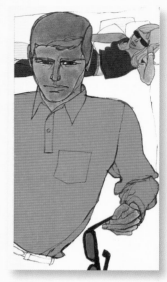

Above Horrors! – Men were starting to wear coloured shirts!

Left October 1969 – the average man at the end of the decade. His clothes are far more colourful – note the beige shirt! – and his hair positively shaggy compared to the start of the sixties.

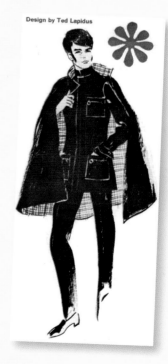

Design by Ted Lapidus

Right Design by Ted Lapidus, February 1968. Few men would wear quite such revolutionary clothes, but nevertheless there had been great changes.

1960

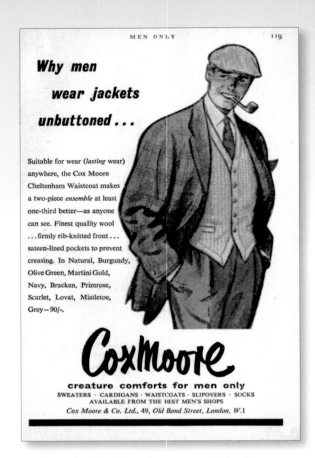
Right Ill-fitting baggy jacket, knitted waistcoat, pipe and flat cap – Mr Britain, March 1960.

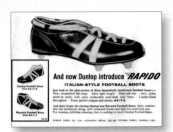

Above Italian styling was the coming thing. Rapido football boot by Dunlop.

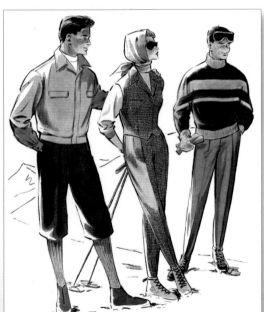

Above Foreign holidays, and even skiing holidays were increasingly available to ordinary Britons. There they would see continental styling, and began to want it.

In the 1950s Pierre Cardin had become the first haute couture designer to produce a ready-to-wear collection for women. For this he was banished from the Couture-Creation list of the Fédération Française de la Couture. However, the idea proved a great success and was widely copied by other couturiers, leading to his rapid reinstatement. In 1960 he produced his first ready-to-wear collection of menswear.

The collection was dubbed the 'Youth line' or the 'Cylinder line'. The latter name referred to the long, slim shaping. The collection owed a great deal to the style which had developed in Britain featuring tweed and worsteds. Jackets were narrow-shouldered, fitted at the waist and had high sleeve holes. Trousers were high-waisted and flat-fronted. The most important creations were round-necked, tail-less jackets, which were made in corduroy for winter, and striped cotton for summer. These would be taken up by The Beatles and become known the world over as Beatle jackets.

On the streets, however, men's clothing was still very much stuck in the 1950s with the 'cardy' [cardigan] perhaps the most informal part of most men's wardrobes.

The old, drab, shapeless style of men's suits was being updated. **Men Only** magazine predicted that *'The trend in suits will be to the slim line and the athletic look. The jacket will have a slightly shorter collar with longer jacket lapels which will also be narrower. The back of the jacket will be straight-hanging to create this 1960 husky,* *athletic look. The advantage of the longer and narrower lapels is that they give the wearer the appearance of added height.*

'Continuing the suit silhouette downwards, the trousers will remain narrow. They will be finished with a smaller turn-up. This will give added length to the legs. The trend in patterns is to checked materials for jackets and trousers, and for the two-piece sports suit.'

The tie had traditionally been a man's one permitted piece of colour in an otherwise drab outfit, and this trend continued. The fashion for not wearing waistcoats or, in the summer, jumpers meant that ties were made far longer than they had been, now reaching down to just above the waist instead of mid-chest. In the first half of the 1960s the fashion was towards the 'slim Jim' tie, which accentuated the slimline look so fashionable in suits, jackets and trousers. In March **Men Only** described this process, *'Although some men prefer the 3 ½ in. width, the most fashionable tie now measures 3 in. wide. There is also a trend to straight-ended ties as distinct from pointed ends. These can be even narrower, say 2 in.'*

1961

In 1961, following the success of Cardin's show the previous year, the clothing manufacturer Brill produced a complete line of men's ready-to-wear clothing designed by Cardin. Although they might be ready-to-wear, they were still well beyond the pocket of most men, who had to buy their clothes from cheaper outlets.

The slow but sure movement towards a less-formal fashion for men was best seen in lightweight suits and casual wear. **Men Only** commented that *'Sales of lightweight suits are accelerating because men like the feel, the finish, and the freedom of action they offer. Two grades from Italy, the Marzotte and the Lido, possess all the most popular lightweight characteristics – the styling is*

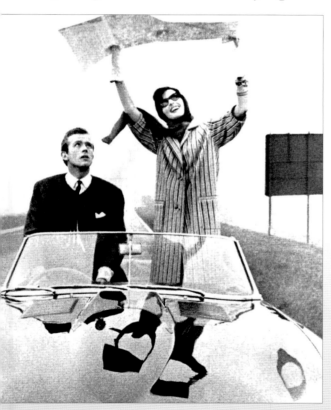

pure British, tailored with true Italian understanding of these modern cloths. With hand-finished buttonholes, shoulders, and collars, they feature two breast pockets and two styles of trousers, conventional and

slim. The interlinings are all-wool canvas.'

While for general leisurewear *'Lightweight knitted garments are now being specially styled for the summer months. Sweater shirts are available in either wool or man-made fibres such as nylon and Courtelle. Double-knit fabrics are being used for lightweight club jackets, which can be worn when there's a slight nip in the air on those cooler summer evenings.*

'The clear, crisp look is the new mood of casual wear for the weekend. White has been the obvious colour choice and is now being featured in both shirts and cotton knitwear for this year. The white sweater finds ready acceptance with blue slacks and check shirts. White -- once the province of tennis players and the ladies, will be particularly popular in many of the younger man's casual styles.'

In May **Men Only** informed its readers that *'Tradition has taken its last, deep breath – and the lightweight suit is now established in this country. The average man's enthusiasm for lightweights resulted in more of them being bought in 1960 than in any previous year. They ranged in price from ten to 16 guineas. The time is coming when every man will have a lightweight suit in his wardrobe. He will make his choice in 1961 from a colourful range of new lightweights. To date, the colour chart reads – light navy, coffee, natural, and grey. Most men show a preference for navy and grey, claiming that they are more in keeping with the business world. And the weight? Most men in this country do not want the feather-weight styles as worn in America. This country's climate favours anything upwards of 9 and 10 ounces, a lighter weight by six or seven ounces than some of the suits worn in the past.'*

In September **Men Only** described the latest suit: *'A new double-breasted suit for autumn and winter has only two buttons. This, with the narrow lapels and no turn-ups, gives it a slim line more usually*

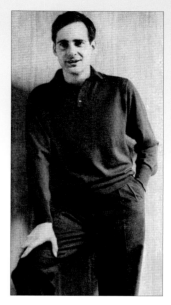

Above *Casual wear became brighter and more stylish, like the sweater shirt – this one in Courtelle from May.*

Left *June 1961. A taste of things to come – Cardin suit, of the type later made famous by the Beatles, worn with a slim Jim tie, a glamorous companion and a Jag – what more could a man ask.*

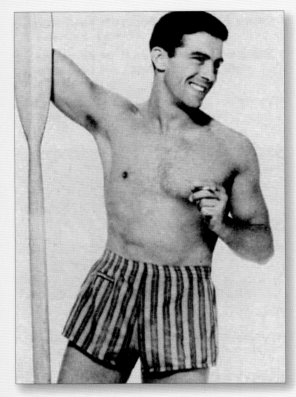

Above Boxer shorts for beach wear were the latest thing, these in nylon with a plastic zip on the pocket. May 1961.

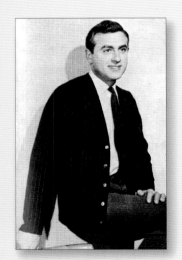

Above Even the humble cardigan evolved into the 'club jacket'. This example from May 1961.

associated with single-breasted suits.'

The magazine also described the new fashion in shirts; *'Patterned shirts are coming back, and the most marked trend is to stripes. Many of the leading shirt manufacturers are featuring very bold Bengal stripes in their autumn ranges. These are essentially for the businessman, the man who normally wears a fairly plain dark suit. Colouring of the stripes is generally dark – black, maroon or navy blue, but pastel blues and greys can be obtained in some ranges.'*

In September 1961, the magazine described another change in ties; *'One result of the striped-shirt trend will be a return to plain ties. Regimental and club ties can be worn, but only if they have a small motif.'*

The raincoat has always been essential in Britain and, like the overcoat, it reflected the move towards the slimline look. **Men Only** described the latest trend in an October issue: *'The problem of keeping warm out of doors without having to wear heavy outer clothing this winter will be partly solved by "foam backs". These are knitted or woven fabrics on the back of which a thin layer of foam plastic has been laminated. Foambacked knitted fabrics have been used for lightweight casual jackets, windcheaters and car coats. Foambacked woven fabrics have been used for ski-jackets, raincoats, and overcoats. Their advantage: they are warm without being heavy. Overcoats, for example, are being made from tweeds which until now have been used for suits and sportscoats. They can be dry-cleaned.*

'You will shortly be able to buy cotton gabardine raincoats which are foambacked, also golf jackets. Another foambacked raincoat is in cotton cloth which is water repellent. It can be washed or dry-cleaned.'

The trench coat style was replaced by a slim, short-look, unbelted coat, sometimes with the buttons hidden. Overcoats followed the same line, becoming ever shorter. **Men Only** in July declared that *'the sartorial revolution continues. The latest attack is on rainwear. That cumbersome full-length heavy wool gabardine raincoat in a fawn shade and with a belt that is seldom kept in place has been finally overthrown. Successor to those gabardines (and the slovenly-looking plastic macs) are the new short-length weather coats now being styled in a variety of hardwearing materials, lively colours, and even livelier linings. The Annadillo weathercoat in BriNylon with a Botany wool fleece lining in colourful checks is an example of this new short cut to style. It features a roll collar, turn back cuffs and leather buttons. In the now fashionable finger-tip length, it retails around the ten guinea mark. The Borderer is the name given to another of these short jacket coats. With slant pockets, leather buttons and side vents, it, too, has a shawl collar in wool and a detachable fleece lining for the cooler days and evenings.'*

In October **Men Only** commented that *'the leisure cardigan has almost become the leisure-jacket. Byford have transformed the "ordinary warm woolly", into a fashion garment. Their model for this winter is called Chalfont. Style points to note are the black ribbed cuffs and deep, shield-shaped collar. The material is a fancy jacquard jersey. Colour combinations include graphite and grey, raisin and heron blue, black and olive, greenfinch and off-white. To retail at £5 5s.*

'Another stylish example of the leisure jacket, or club jacket as it is now called,

comes from the Scottish knitwear house of McCallum and Craigie. The Kintyre is available in charcoal, with roll collar and leather buttons. Retail price is £7 19s 6d.'

In September the magazine reported that: '*The trend to more comfort and less weight in evening dress continues. With fewer men wearing white tie and tails, the black tie and dinner jacket is undergoing a number of significant style changes. The single-breasted dinner jacket in the shawl-collar style promises to remain the most fashionable for this autumn and winter. There will be greater variety in cloths, with mohair worsted and Terylene worsteds providing dinner jackets that are much lighter in weight and more comfortable to wear.*

'*We shall also see the return of the cummerbund. Rocola are making them in*

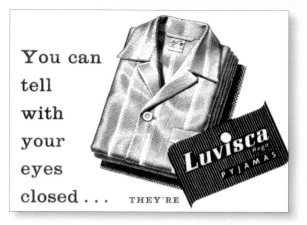

Oriental-style brocade with maroon, deep blue, black or gold ground colours. A more simple design has air force blue, red or grey for the main colour. Both will be sold with matching bow-ties for about £1 15s. Plain pure-silk cummerbunds in black or maroon will cost about £1 15s; with matching bow-ties around £2 2s. Dress shirts, too, will be lighter in weight.'

With the coming of summer in July, **Men Only** described the latest beach fashions. '*Brief, briefer, briefest…That's the trend in swimwear. For this summer Jantzen have brought out a very brief Continental-styled trunk, which will undoubtedly be popular with younger men for both its streamlined look and masculine eye-appeal. In plain, gay colours, or in wavy-striped or checked nylon, this brief style will certainly bring a Continental flavour to any British resort. Colours to choose from in swim trunks this year include peacock blues, vivid reds, greens and deep browns.*

'*Any pattern with a stripe in it, either for boxer shorts or swim trunks, it would seem, will be fashionable for the swimmer this summer. Continental styling has influenced the 1961 swim trunk ranges of a number of houses. The trend is to briefer swim trunks, and shorts are also being styled shorter. The boxer short is not affected. This versatile beach wear garment serves the dual role of a swim short and play short after the swim. Quick-drying nylon is a favourite fabric.*'

Left Men's pyjamas had changed little in design, but like most other clothes, could now be got in the latest man-made fibres, easy to wash and iron – a boon for the batchelor. December 1961.

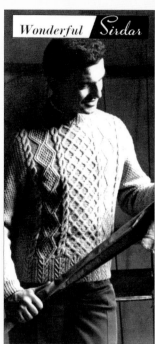

Above For many men, an Arran sweater was about as far as casual clothes went.

Far left December 1961 – for most men the question was whether to a wear white shirt, or to be daring with a striped shirt.

1962

In January, **Men Only** advised its readers that *'Lightweight cloths will predominate in the ready-to-wear suit ranges for spring '62, but the stress will be on lighter weights in the 9 oz to 13 oz range, with a growing emphasis on blends of different fibres, particularly of Terylene and other man-made fibres with wool. Patterns will concentrate on small neat checks, overchecks and fancy weaves. Suitings will be darker, but with admixtures of brighter colours. Blacks, browns and the heavier shades of bronze will be lightened*

would spawn a look which would later be associated with 'dodgy' salesmen, but at the time was seen as the height of cool – the short car coat, often worn with an open necked shirt and cravat, flat cap and, of course, driving gloves.

Men Only again: *'The Sweater Jacket designed by Hardy Amies for Hepworths is in a black /gold check all-wool tweed, intended for wearing over a chunky sweater and not over a sports jacket or the jacket of a two-piece suit. This "shortie" has raglan shoulders, vertical pockets, four front buttons and one on the cuff. About 10 guineas.'*

Terylene was one of the new man-made yarns which, blended with other fabrics, made lightweight textiles that were as easy-care as the new drip-dry shirts. In 1962 a new fabric for 'sports trousers' was brought out, a blend of 67 per cent Terylene and 33 per cent cotton. These new blends had several advantages; they could be washed or dry-cleaned and were inexpensive; the trousers costing only £2 19s 6d.

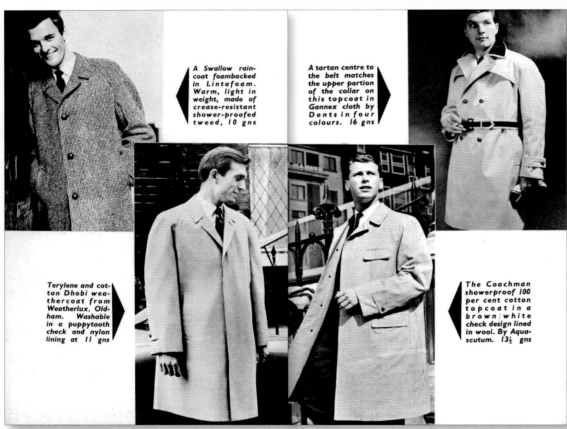

A Swallow rain-coat foambacked in Lintafoam. Warm, light in weight, made of crease-resistant shower-proofed tweed, 10 gns

A tartan centre to the belt matches the upper portion of the collar on this topcoat in Gannex cloth by Dents in four colours. 16 gns

Terylene and cotton Dhobi wea-thercoat from Weatherlux, Oldham. Washable in a puppytooth check and nylon lining at 11 gns

The Coachman showerproof 100 per cent cotton topcoat in a brown/white check design lined in wool. By Aquascutum. 13½ gns

by greens and gold, with olive and mustard the favourite shades.'

Increasing car ownership meant that motoring clothing became a serious look. In 1951 less than 15 per cent of families had a car, but this had almost doubled by the start of the 1960s, and the figure would be over 50 per cent by the end of the decade. This

One tailoring house carried out a survey in 1962 to find out what men spent on their clothes. It discovered that the man in the £2000-a-year-plus income bracket had about 13 suits in his wardrobe, counting tails, dinner jacket, sports jacket and trousers, and topcoats each as a separate suit, representing a capital value of about £400. These would last him for some time, as men bought on average one and two-thirds suits a year, representing a turn-around time of about eight years. Unsurprisingly, a man would buy the suits himself from his tailor, whereas his wife would usually buy his socks and underwear and, less commonly, his shirts.

Most formal shirts were still bought with detachable collars, and this led to a new fashion. **Men Only** reported in January that *'the trend to bold-patterned shirts, especially in Bengal stripes has resulted in striped shirts with white attached collars. These white-collar jobs are appearing with increasing frequency and are a logical development from the city habit of wearing detachable white collars with striped shirts.*

'John Church, the Manchester shirt-making firm who have a number of bold Bengal stripes in their new ranges, have introduced one shirt in this style. The collar is in the contemporary cut-away shape.

'A new "Prime-fit" shirt by Famox Ltd features a white collar attached to a striped shirt and plain white cuffs – further evidence, if it were necessary, that in the field of design the British shirt manufacturers are some of the most lively and original thinkers in the men's clothing and outfitting trade.'

As the article mentions the fashionable collar now had shorter points; in February the magazine reported another collar innovation, this time in casual-shirt collars; *'Shirt makers are finding a trend to the button-down rounded collar. The latest addition to the Van Heusen Collarite range has a casual button-down rounded collar and rounded single cuffs to link or button. To sell at £2 5s in colours or £1 19s 6d in white.'*

In April the magazine noted that *'Bow-tie addicts will be interested in two new shirts, both of which have concealed buttons to give an unbroken line down the centre*

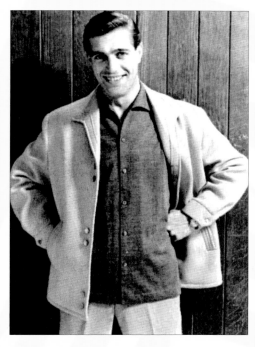

front. One, by Scott-Ward, features a new blend of 25 per cent silk and 75 per cent Terylene. The fly-front style allows more buttons to be used than normally. Collar and cuffs are stiffened and the shirt can be drip-dried. Price is 4 guineas. A casual shirt with the same type of fastening is the 9-Pin by Activity. Made in non-iron cotton with subdued broken-check design, it has a permanently-stiffened collar, and a breast pocket. Made in blue or maroon, the 9-Pin costs £1 7s 6d with half-sleeves, £1 12s 6d with long.'

Men Only complained that *'if topcoats get any shorter we'll soon be wearing them as jackets. Already they're being called Sweater Jackets or Car Jackets, and the idea behind this short cut to coat styling, it would seem, is to do away with the sports jacket in cooler months for out-of-doors casual occasions.'* The car coat continued to be the popular style for men throughout the 1960s. It was so named because when getting into a car you weren't inconvenienced by sitting on the tails of the coat, something that was both uncomfortable and caused creases.

Meanwhile, *'The trend to "string" underwear continues. Activity Textiles are now supplying this modern and hygienic underwear suitable to the changeable weather because its "air pockets" provide insulation against both heat and cold. The many features of this new fine mesh "string" (over 35 air pockets to the square inch) include a particularly soft texture, tailored appearance, comfortable close fit and lightness in wear. New "string" singlet-vests and centre-front trunks retail at 8s 6d each in all sizes.'*

Left *Courtelle single jersey leisure jacket with foam plastic backing, washable and drip-dry. February 1962.*

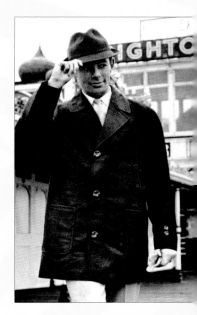

Above *Shortie coat from April 1962. The shortie, especially in the form of the car coat, would be one of the staples of older men's clothing in the sixties.*

1963

That year the cinemas showed **Beau Fashion**, a Pathé news short which looked at men's fashions, starting with a catwalk parade which included such manly characters as motor-racing driver Bruce McLaren, footballer Bobby Smith and cricketer Alec Bedser. The commentary talked about mens' suits – *'Too often in the past middle age reserve kept it confined to charcoal greys and drab designs, but that too is changing. British reserve is taking a*

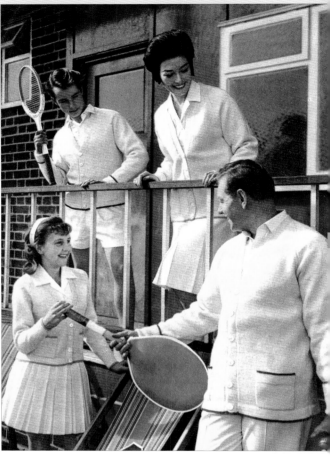

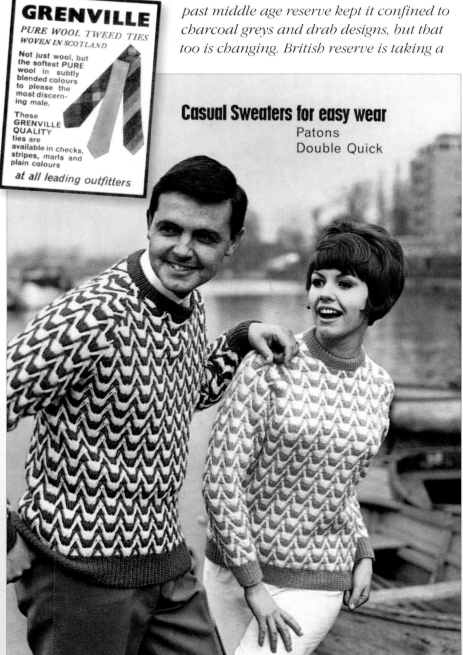

beating, colour and cut is on the warpath. A path which began with the post-war demob suit.

'The reaction against such a mess resulted in the Italian style. Italy was the young man's benefactor – it gave him everything, a hairstyle, a suit, even shoes. The dandy has returned with a whole new range of colourful wool cloth that has bid adieu to the drabness; that has said goodbye to the browns and blues and greys and encouraged men to buy. But colour-woven wool has inspired more than the urge to buy. It's inspired a design that is catching on with amazing speed – it has inspired the peacock era; suits of two matching cloths that differ but harmonise excitingly.'

Left Matching leisure sweaters were just the thing for couples – the fashion would slowly grow into unisex clothing.

The film went on to list some interesting reasons '*for this sudden switch to a man's world of elegance and style include the broader outlook induced by foreign travel, the fact that smokeless zones are encouraging gayer colours, that cloths of lighter weight have meant new shapes, that dry cleaning has given clothes a shorter life, but perhaps all these are subservient to the stars of pop music who have spread more than anything the cult of dressing differently.*'

By the start of the decade the influence of American music and youth fashion was in decline; rock-and-roll music was increasingly linked to delinquency and its appeal was being usurped by 'pop' music. A particularly British sound was coming from the north; it was soon christened 'Merseybeat' and featured groups such as Gerry and the Pacemakers, Freddie and the Dreamers and The Beatles.

In May the single 'From Me To You' by The Beatles reached number one where it remained for seven weeks. 'Beatlemania' swept the country and their highly individual dress style was widely copied. In 1961 they had dressed in the rock-and-roll look of T-shirts and leather motorcycle jackets; now under the influence of their manager Brian Epstein, they wore sharp suits with white shirts and ties, but all in the most modern styles, like their Pierre Cardin-inspired collarless jackets (actually made by Dougie Millings), soon re-named Beatle jackets. These were best set off by a high, round-collared shirt, kept rigidly up the neck by a buttoned tab. The most fashionable of these were in paisley, although for work plain colours or stripes were often preferred. These would be worn with slim Jim ties, Cuban-heeled Chelsea winklepicker boots and, of course, 'mop-top' hairstyles.

As the Pathé newsreel stated, these were all copied and became highly fashionable. People could now buy Beatle suits and jackets, Nehru jackets, shirts with rounded collars, Cuban-heeled boots and even Merseybeat wigs.

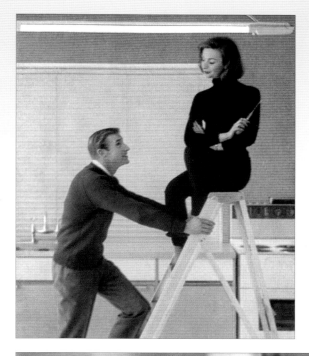

Above *The slimline look in the form of narrower trousers and a well-fitting sweater.*

Below *The clothes are the same, knitted waistcoat and tie, but men are discovering colour.*

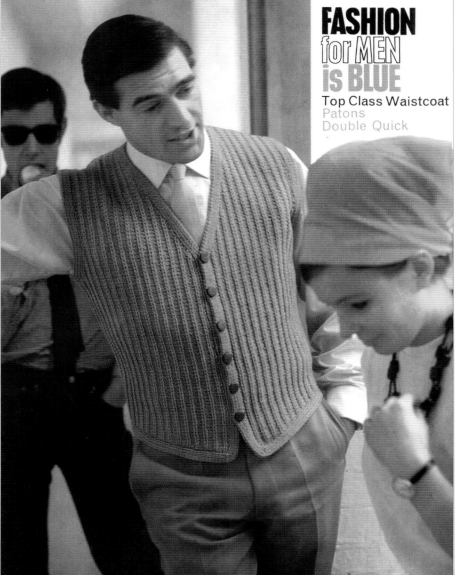

FASHION for MEN is BLUE

Top Class Waistcoat
Patons
Double Quick

1964

By 1964 the look which was to be the epitome of the swinging 1960s was firmly established. The Beatles were taking the United States by storm, and the youth look had become unassailable as manufacturers began to wake up to the fact that Britain and all things British were now seen as 'Fab', and highly sought after.

The music scene continued to influence male fashion, which, via the Mods, became such a vibrant phenomenon that even women's magazines begin to cover it; a situation that had almost never happened before. For example, **Boyfriend Annual** that summer reported that *'strictly for boys – so hands off, girls — is a reversible poplin jacket in beige – which is also made in a more expensive needlecord – and sells for around £6. The one our model is wearing*

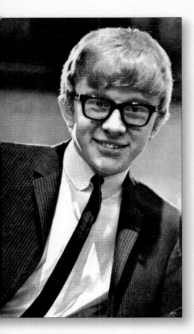

Below *Tab-collar shirt, a very slim Jim tie, and a lightweight suit with a very sixties colar, May 1964.*

Right *The dandy is back. Notice especially the longer button down collar, and the glimpse of Edwardian styling in the bowler. December 1965.*

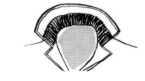

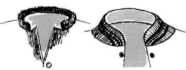

Above *A selection of collars for fashionable casual jackets.*

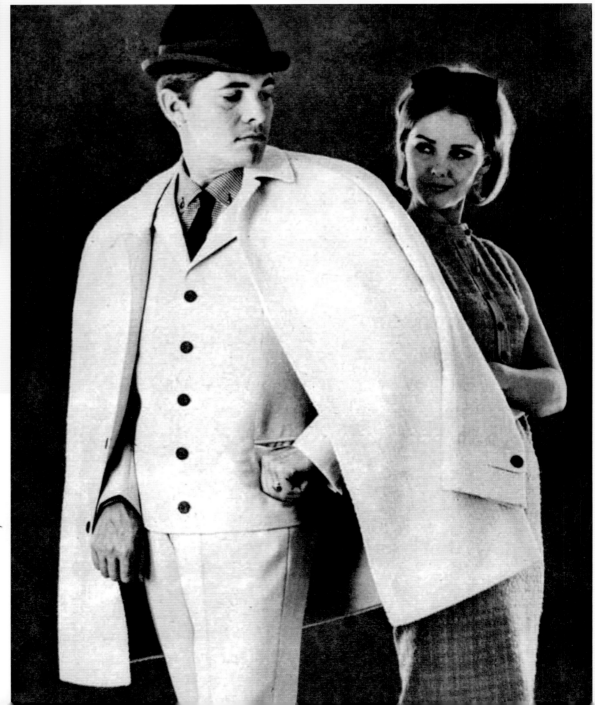

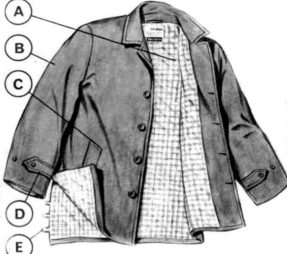
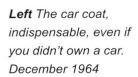
Left The car coat, indispensable, even if you didn't own a car. December 1964

Below left The hair and tight trousers could be from the fifties, but the short collar, tie and short jersey top make this 1964.

Below right Many fashions of the time were a real fusion of the late 1950s and early 1960s; note the bang up to date Beatle-necked jacket and button-down shirt, but the very fifties hairstyle with quiff.

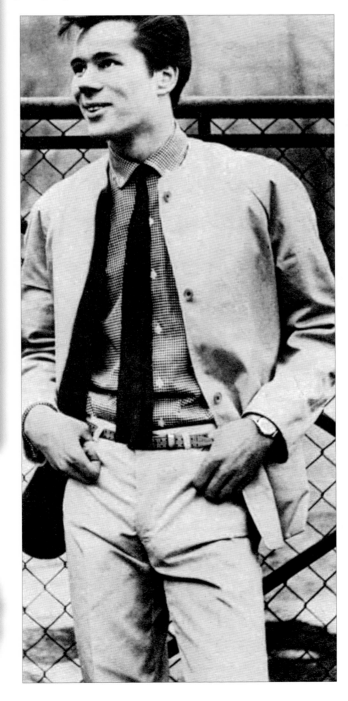

reverses to navy blue for your evening date, so you'd better make sure you're dressed up enough to look as good as your boy will in this. For, despite its casual look, with a collar and tie it's dressy enough for the smartest place. Note the collar on this jacket – similar to our cardigans, girls.

The polo shirt in bright primary colours was all the fashion, worn with jeans if possible; if you were a Mod, who started the fashion, these would have to be a Fred Perry shirt and Levi jeans.

1965

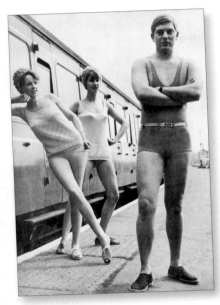

Pierre Cardin's ready-to-wear men's clothing had boomed. It was estimated that more than half a million men were now wearing his clothes. Yet on the horizon a new look, or even a movement, was forming. Hippies, who had sprung from small beginnings in San Francisco, began to be seen in London. It was a ground-breaking philosophy in fashion terms, rejecting the overt consumerism of Carnaby Street and the King's Road, but in 1965 it was still in its infancy. For most fashionable people the pursuit of that fashion still meant spending as much of one's disposable income as possible.

That August The Beatles played at New York's Shea Stadium, wearing very military style jackets, of the sort worn by British soldiers in the tropics in the late nineteenth century, with patch pockets, epaulettes, and most distinctly, an upright collar, otherwise known as a Mandarin collar. The style took off, becoming known as the Nehru jacket after the Indian prime minister. Later versions accentuated the plain, uncluttered line by losing the epaulettes and dispensing with pockets (or at least none were visible). The style with its overtones of futurism would remain popular throughout the rest of the decade.

In 1965 the 'Kipper tie', invented by Michael Fish, became all the rage. The name was both a description of the very broad tie

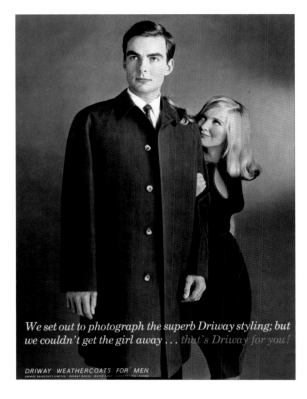

We set out to photograph the superb Driway styling; but we couldn't get the girl away . . . that's Driway for you!

DRIWAY WEATHERCOATS FOR MEN

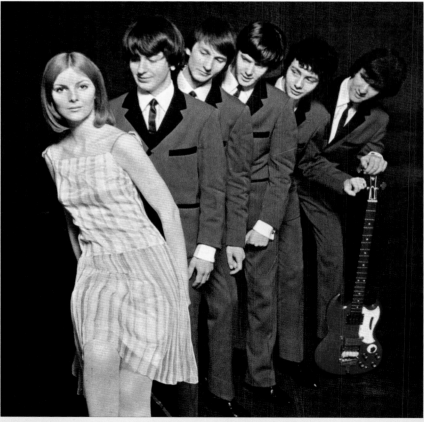

and a play on its designer's name. Kippers became the easel on which increasingly bold and bright patterns could be showcased.

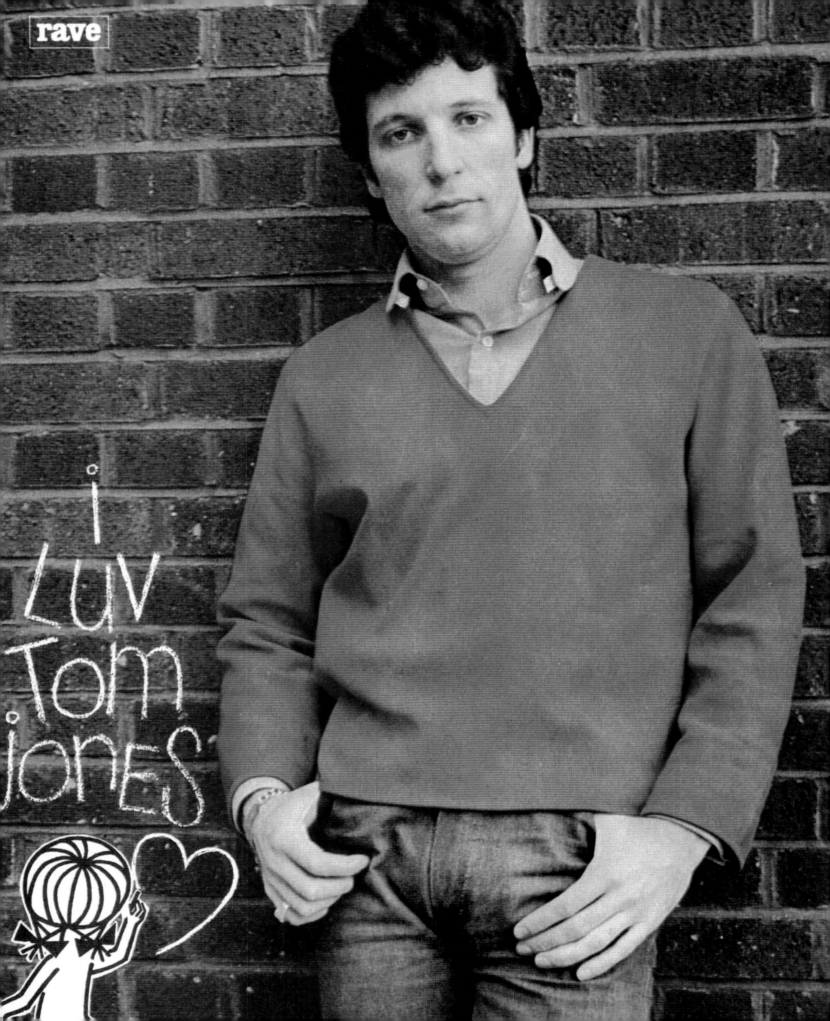

1966

In Paris five designers: Andre Bardot, Jose Camps, Socrate, Gaston Waltener and Max Evzeline, known collectively as the Groupe des Cinq (Group of Five) were trying to create the idea of haute couture for men, with patchy success. They were applauded in the fashion press for their attempts to liven up menswear, but condemned for their attempts to get men to carry handbags, which they called 'man cases'. The reality was that they were too late; Pierre Cardin's ready-to-wear lines had already covered much of their ground, and the idea of livening up menswear was now almost old hat on the streets where the peacock revolution was in full swing. Clothing which would, just a few years earlier, have put its wearer in danger of being beaten up for being effeminate was now increasingly seen as normal, with the way being led by the Rolling Stones, who became the pet hate figures of establishment types.

Yet in the same year as The Kinks released 'Dedicated Follower of Fashion' the sharply-dressed Mod movement was slowly dying out, to be replaced by the hippy look, and the fashionable drugs shifted from pep pills to cannabis and LSD. This trend was reflected in the name of the King's Road's latest boutique, Granny Takes A Trip. At the same time Michael Fish opened his shop, Mr Fish, in London's Clifford Street which soon became a magnet for London's 'beautiful people'.

Carnaby Street took up a khaki theme that year. Seeking bargains, some canny shoppers descended on the military surplus stores then to be found in most towns. They

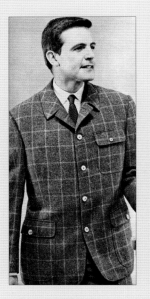

had been discovered by the Mods some years before, who shopped there for parkas and other cold-weather wear for use on their scooters. Now buyers scoured them for other fashionable wear, and accidentally a whole new fashion was born. **The Observer** magazine would later describe it: '*Hanging*

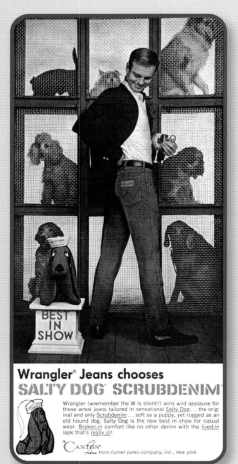

Wrangler® Jeans chooses
SALTY DOG SCRUBDENIM

Wrangler (wremember the W is silent!) wins wild applause for these wreal jeans tailored in sensational Salty Dog...the original and only Scrubdenim...soft as a puppy, yet rugged as an old hound dog. Salty Dog is the new best in show for casual wear. Broken-in comfort like no other denim with the lived-in look that's really in!

CANTON from turner jones company, inc., new york

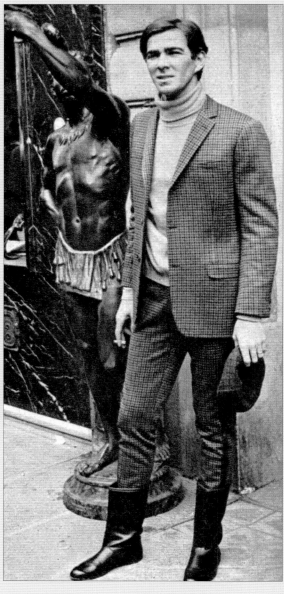

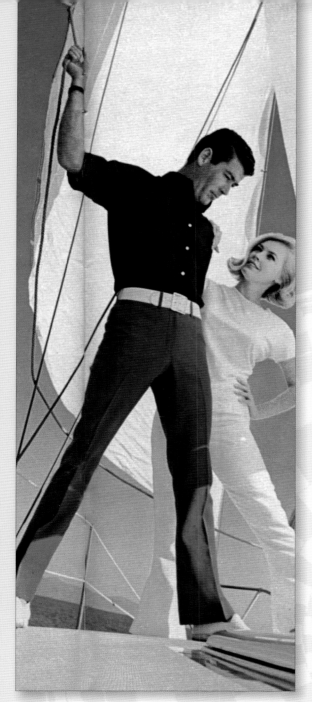

the lure was too great; not only were the uniforms smart, being covered in the kind of tassels, braid and velvet that was very much part of the peacock revolution, they were also part of the surreal Edwardian look which was beginning to permeate the whole fashion/design scene. Added to this, there was definitely an element of establishment-baiting in wearing one; doing so made retired colonels in Tunbridge Wells almost explode with indignation, and the press had a field day. That October, in what became something of a cause célèbre, Mazin Zeki, 18, of Muswell Hill, was charged *'that not being a person in her Majesty's military forces, he did wear part of a uniform of the Scots Guards without her Majesty's permission'* on Holborn Viaduct. He was, however, conditionally discharged.

The **Observer** reported; ' *"If Army discipline and Army haircuts could be put on with the uniform it might be a good thing for these young men," says Major de Zulueta for the Brigade of Guards. Are they still pressing for arrests? "Look what happened when we did," says a spokesman gloomily. But they needn't give up hope. Under the London Waiting and Loading Regulations of 1961 it is forbidden to wear "fancy dress within three miles of Charing Cross".'*

on the rails of the same shops were scarlet tunics, bell-bottoms and waistcoats with high Prussian collars. With tailored waists and bright colours, cloaks and gold trimmings, these were clothes to cut a dash in. Right in tune with the new era of the peacock, they provided instant dandyism, high fashion without too much imagination, or too much expense.'

The latest fashion was old Edwardian-style military dress uniforms, although at that time you were in danger of being arrested for wearing the Queen's uniform without proper reason. However, for many

Left April 1966 – just a hint of flare on the trousers. Notice also – it's hard to miss it – the wide white belt.

Below Fun fur, October 1966. In this particular colour it had overtones of a giant teddy bear.

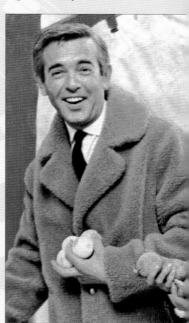

Left A range of fashionable 'sleep suits' from April 1966.

1967

Far right *Lightweight worsted-and-mohair suit by Austin Reed.*

Large floral prints were the latest fashion. **Titbits** magazine that July told its readers that *'If the girls are asking; "Where have all the flowers gone?" the boys know. They ought to. They're wearing them. For suddenly it's OK for men to wear clothes that look like seed packets or the more gaudy kind of floral wallpapers.'* Jackets made from floral curtain or upholstery materials cost 12 guineas.

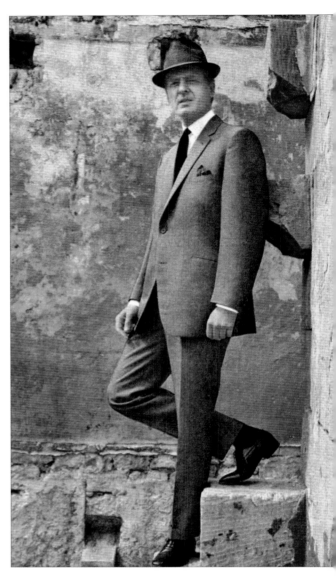

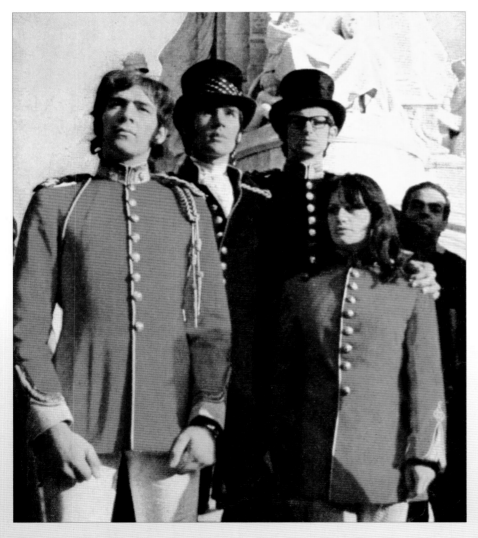

Above *March 1967 and old military uniforms are all the rage, much to the fury of retired colonels.*

The military uniform look had become all the rage. I Was Lord Kitchener's Valet, owned by Ian Fisk, was described as *'London's first second-hand boutique for kinky, period and military gear.'* It was situated *'at the* wrong end of the Portobello Road in London'*, and was doing a roaring trade in slightly altered, and therefore legal, ex-military jackets. In March a new branch was opened in Wardour Street, Soho. One of their best sellers that summer was a brass-buttoned bush jacket in fawn cotton drill, costing 30s.

The **Observer** magazine covered the new look: *'Where else, if you fancy that sort of thing, could you buy a jacket as gilded and well cut as the Royal Fusiliers tunic marked up at £7 10s.! With a bit of work on them – velvet collar and cuffs, a change of buttons – they fetch around 10 guineas, and the modifications may preserve you from*

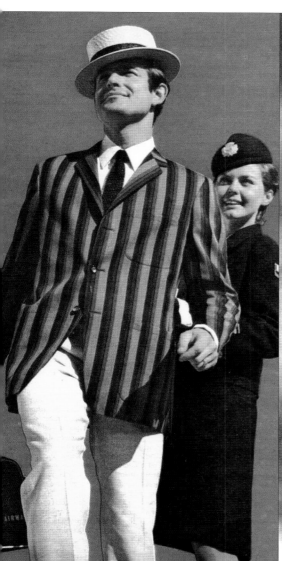

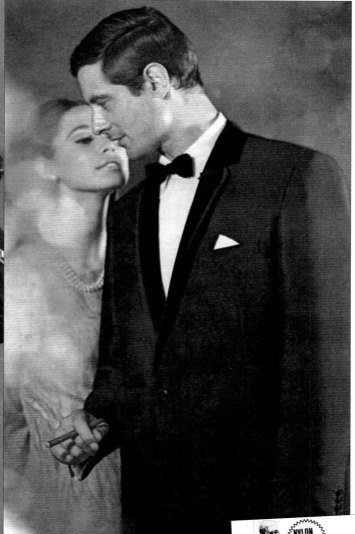

Far left An Edwardian-style outfit with more than a little of the panache that had defined the singer Frankie Vaughan.
Left Hector Powe dinner jacket suit.

Below Space-age style suit from May 1967.

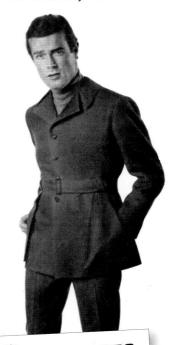

arrest.' One wearer commented, 'Fancy dress, fancy dress for soldiers, that's what it was designed as in the first place. Now they have finished with them and they look good on us. So what! The clothes are cheap, warm and practical and the trousers have lots of pockets to put things in. It's no more subtle than that.'

John Stephen designed his own versions of the military look, including what he called the 'Khartoum' jacket, a variation of the Nehru jacket; single-breasted, pocketless, and with diamond-shaped buttons, it sold for a whopping 30 guineas. The look was certainly spurred on by its adoption by pop groups, for whom its theatrical air was

perfect. Mick Jagger was photographed wearing a very military jacket, with tassels, frogging and braid, but the ultimate accolade came when The Beatles were portrayed in resplendent military-style outfits on the cover of their **Sergeant Pepper's Lonely Hearts Club Band** album that June.

By 1968 the US jacket-maker After Six was even producing a formal version of the Nehru jacket in brocaded silk for evening wear, as well as a range of coloured evening jackets.

Above Tracksuits in July 1967, when almost everybody wearing one was actually doing something sport-related.

1968

That year's smash-hit film, **Bonnie and Clyde**, spawned a fashion look, as young men tried to look like Warren Beatty. The 'gangster' look sent many of them into the second-hand shops where demob suits were snapped up, as well as trilby and homburg hats, and even correspondence shoes and spats. Alternative variations were dark pin-stripe suits with a black shirt and white tie, or a large cloth cap and a Fair Isle pullover. In June **Men Only** reported that *'the younger generation of at least relatively honest and respectable Teenagers are coasting along on the revivalist 'Thirties fashions of Bonnie and Clyde. Thus the Chalk Stripes, the shady brimmed Fedora hats, and the wildly coloured Kipper ties of the Gangster era are acquiring an innocent Teenage naivete just as the Racketeers who seek such a projection are leaving them off.'*

As the decade wore on, so conventions, long ago smashed by the young and fashionable, were also breaking down among older, more conservative males. There had been many variations on the suit, depending on the time, function, or place that it was to be worn – the morning suit, lounge suit, town suit, dinner jacket, business suit, etc. Now the strict lines between them were wearing away, as reported in **Men Only** that June: *'With prices of almost everything boosted by the last Budget – in the wrong direction – the fashionable man is forced to cut down on the number of new additions to his wardrobe. So Savile Row tailors, Lew Rose, have come up with a solution – three suits for the price of one, i.e. the "All Purpose" suit. This outfit can be worn for the office and everyday wear, a drink at the local pub or an evening at the Hilton*

simply by changing shirt and tie. At a "beat the Budget" price of 24 guineas.'

The use of new man-made fibres continued. **Woman** magazine that April, told its readers that, *'We have been able to buy clothes made in "Crimplene" for some time now, so we know its advantages – fits perfectly, won't wrinkle, can't crease and completely washable! Now it's up to us to tell our men all about it as Guards have just introduced their Lean Line 70 Trouser in "Crimplene": slim fitting with a unique tunnelled belt. Also jackets in "Crimplene"*

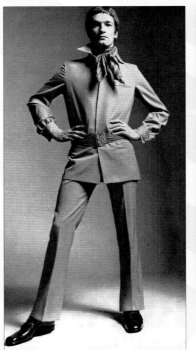
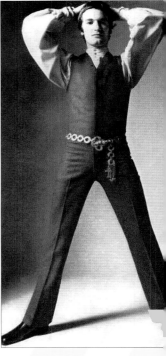

jersey knit cloth, and they can be machine or hand washed and spun dried! Trousers cost from £6.19.6; jackets from £14.14.0.'

Corduroy became popular for both trousers and jackets, the latter either taking the form of windcheaters or cut like normal jackets.

Car coats were still popular, and not only among those who actually owned cars. **Men Only** noted wryly that *'...if there was a car in the garage for every car-coat in the wardrobes throughout Britain, our roads would long ago have seized up in the ultimate jam which doubtless is on the way.'*

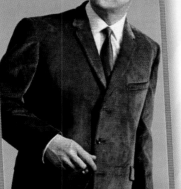

Below *Corduroy jacket.*

Right *October 1968, suit from Worth Esq. the newly formed men's side of the House of Worth.*

Far right *The previous year's retro look led to the romantic look in shirts, with big sleeves, and often big collars, or in this case, a Russian-style collar.*

Opposite page *April 1968 – the end of an era. Men's coloured underpants!*

Under-color-wear.

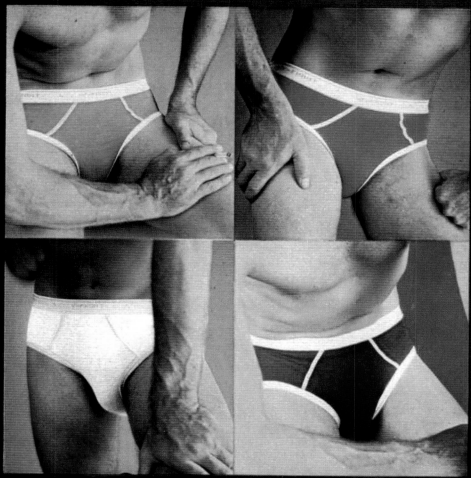

Colour up the action scene with
Slim Guy sports slips.
Liven things up. Add gaiety to masculinity.
You don't have to be a Mr. Muscles.
You do have to be bold.
Jump the gun. Be the first with
Slim Guy Sports slips in pure cotton 6/11d.

Slim Guy
'Y-FRONT'
MADE BY LYLE & SCOTT

1969

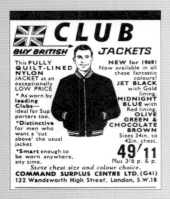

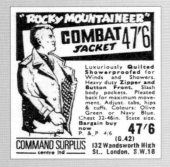

The main influences on menswear were hippy-style ethnic clothing, blended with a flamboyant romanticism. Shirts were loose, with long rounded collars and turned-over cuffs, while man-made fibres were shunned in favour of cotton or cheesecloth. They were rarely worn with a tie; going open-necked with a large pendant on a long chain was far more the fashion, or a jaunty silk neckerchief tied at the side. Alternatively polo-necked shirts were worn Russian-style outside the trousers with a belt over them.

The polo neck jumper was still in fashion, a thin one might be worn under a cardigan, a jumper or a sports jacket, or in colder weather a chunky one under a shortie topcoat.

Velvet was popular, for jackets, suits or trousers and even dress suits, worn with embroidered, pastel-coloured shirts and large, floppy, often velvet, bow ties. Tweed, or wool was popular for sports jackets, sometimes in large checks, sometimes plain. Collars were wider although thin shawl-collars might still be seen on dinner jackets.

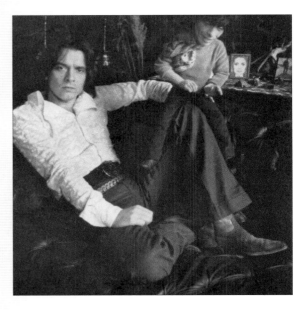

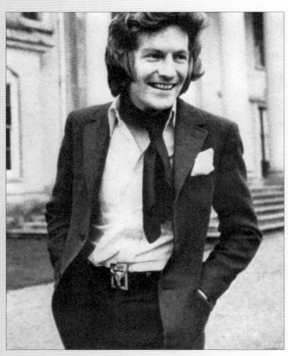

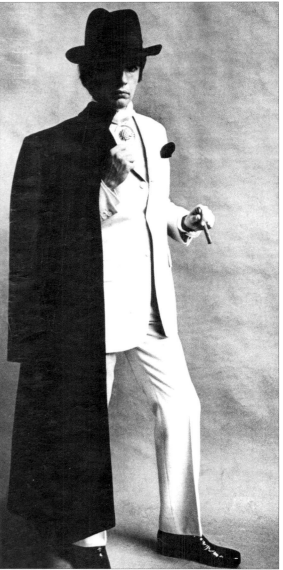

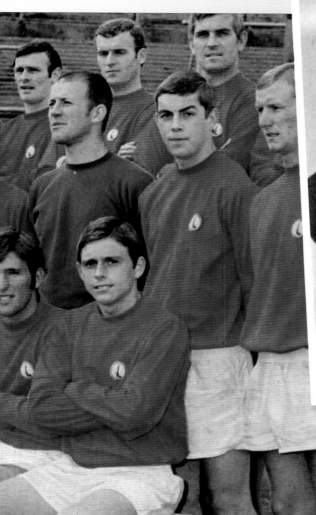

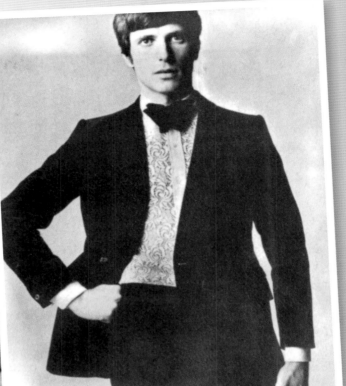

Left *Evening suit, large velvet bowtie and cotton lace evening shirt from John Michael.*

far left *Charlton Athletic, March 1969 with a typical strip of the period – plain-coloured, round necked, heavy shirts, short shorts, thick socks, and where are the advertising logos?*

Below *A bold check on a sports jacket, worn over a polo neck.*

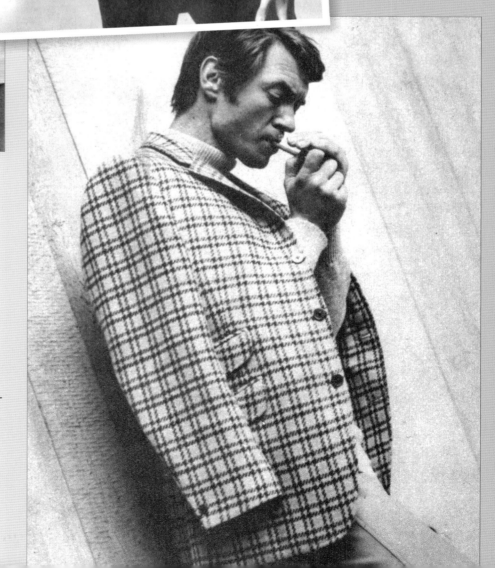

Double-breasted suits were beginning to appear again, often with wing-type collars reminiscent of 1930s style, or such as Napoleon might wear.

Long boots, often in suede, were commonly worn outside the trousers, although flared trousers were becoming popular and were worn outside the boots. Belts were wide, and buckles large and flamboyant.

In topcoats the shortie was still the most popular style, although a very long overcoat might add to a flamboyant suit. Both double- and single-breasted topcoats were popular, as was fur, either as a collar, or as a lining to a leather shortie, often with a military styling. The military look was also present in the combat jacket, either genuine army-surplus or a commercially made example.

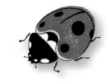

CHILDREN

Both below Chilprufe was most famous for warm children's underwear, but as these ads show, they also produced fairly traditional outer clothes (1961). The short trousers in the first advert. were very up-to-date in September 1963.

Babies' and toddlers' clothes at the start of the 1960s were still very traditional; mostly white with any splash of colour, perhaps in the form of smocking, generally being the standard blue for boys and pink for girls. This situation began to change as man-made fibres brought both washability and bright colour to children's wear, while growing resistance to sexual stereotyping began to make the conventional boy/girl colour scheme seem outmoded. One of the greatest revolutions in babies' clothing

poppers down the front and inside the legs for ease of access. Nappies could be checked and changed quickly and easily.

Toddlers' everyday clothes became more practical and unisex in nature, with first the romper suit, which like the babygrow fitted nicely over a nappy, leading to the dungarees or long trousers, worn with a T-shirt and optional jumper, usually hand-knitted. As ever, children's, and especially baby's, clothes were fertile ground for home-knitters.

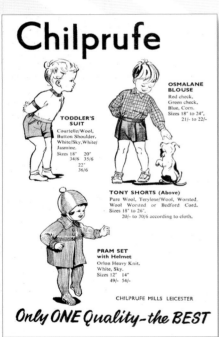

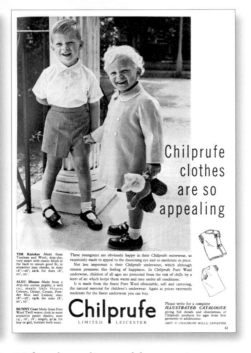

Far right Not all children were dressed in sixties clothes; the party-style frock in the middle could be just about any time post-war. October 1961.

began in 1961 when disposable nappies were introduced into the UK by Pampers. At first sales were low, as people found them quite expensive, and were a little uncertain how best to use them.

The 1960s also saw the introduction of the babygrow, an all-in-one, machine-washable sleepsuit that was fastened by

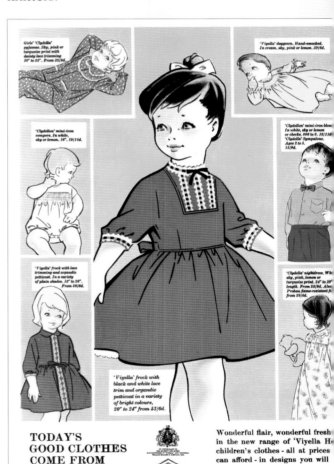

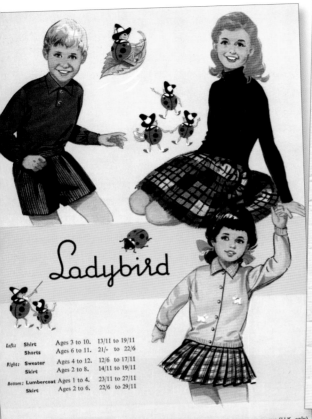

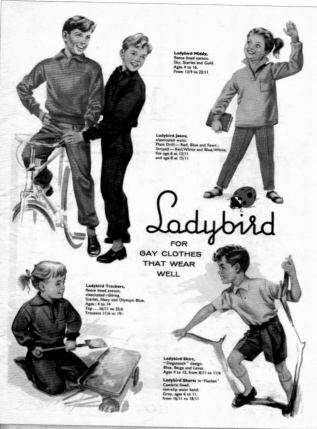

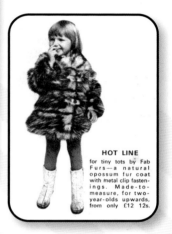

Left *The start of the tracksuit fashion – 'trackers', March 1960, once again, children's clothes are setting the style for the future.*

Far left *The pelmet mini-skirt was not just for adults – October 1964.*

HOT LINE for tiny tots by Fab Furs—a natural opossum fur coat with metal clip fastenings. Made-to-measure, for two-year-olds upwards, from only £12 12s.

Above *Imagine the mess that a jam bun or sticky sweet would make of this fun fur. November 1969.*

For more formal occasions, such as parties or weddings, more traditional clothes were in order. Boys would be dressed in shorts, shirts and ties (usually bow ties), while girls would wear party frocks, often in velvet, usually with lace frills. Both would probably be clad in ankle socks and often sandals. In December 1968 **Woman's Realm** told its readers that the *'Traditional look of velvet trousers and white frill-edged shirt looks great on a mod little boy. And, with weddings in mind; it's a super outfit for a page boy, too!'* As the 1960s progressed, girls' frocks would almost universally be of the smock type, and the ankle socks would be replaced by woolly tights, either ribbed or lacy but still usually white, in a reflection of adult fashion trends.

This blurring of the distinctions between mother's and daughter's fashions was especially marked with the junior age group. Previously girls' clothes had usually progressed from junior to teenage to adult,

but now the fashion was for a youthful look, and the focus changed to teenage fashions.

These teenage fashions also looked good on younger girls, and the various miniskirts, knitted dresses, white knitted tights etc. all saw service as children's wear. Only the older look of the midi-dress, and especially the maxi, failed to take off for children.

This same look, however, did not work so well with boys, although long trousers certainly became the norm from a much earlier age. Previously boys did not generally go into long trousers before their twelfth birthday, but this age now moved to about eight or nine, and often they took the form of jeans for less formal wear. The boy's cap, almost universally worn in the 1950s in the shape of a school cap or Wolf Cub cap, rapidly disappeared in the first few years of the 1960s as going bareheaded became the norm for men.

One new fashion was perfect for children. The rise in the popularity of winter holidays

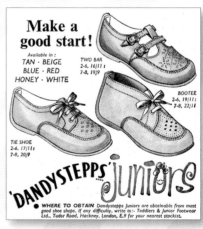

Make a good start!

Available in : TAN · BEIGE BLUE · RED HONEY · WHITE

TWO BAR 2-6, 16/11 7-8, 19/9

BOOTEE 2-6, 19/11 7-8, 22/11

TIE SHOE 2-6, 17/11 7-8, 20/9

'DANDYSTEPPS' **juniors**

● WHERE TO OBTAIN Dandystepps Juniors are obtainable from most good shoe shops. If any difficulty, write to:- Toddlers & Junior Footwear Ltd., Tudor Road, Hackney, London, E.9 for your nearest stockist.

Above *Toddler's shoes – the sandals were a classic style, worn right up to the early teens. April 1963.*

Right As with adults, girls wore shift dresses, which could be converted to trouser suits by the addition of matching trousers, in this case 'bell bottoms in ripple nylon or stretch terry'. November 1969.

Below A children's classic – the duffel coat, October 1964.

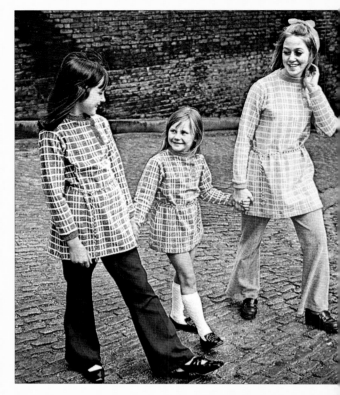

had introduced the anorak as a weatherproof 'action' coat. It proved remarkably adaptable to children's use, and would become ever more popular as the decade wore on, slowly replacing first the macintosh, and then the duffel coat, although both remained in use.

School uniform was one of the last bastions most strongly defended by the traditionalists. For secondary school boys it had hardly changed for at least twenty years, and consisted of a wool blazer in school colours, often with a contrasting piping around the edge and on the lip of the pockets, with the school badge woven onto the breast pocket. This would normally be worn with long trousers, sometimes flannels, a school tie (usually diagonal stripes), shirt (often grey in winter, and white in summer), a jumper in the school colours and black leather shoes. It was common for the socks to come in a specified school colour also, as would the school raincoat. Just about the only changes to this in the early 1960s were that, in most schools, the cap was optional, and therefore rarely worn, and few of the younger secondary boys wore shorts.

For girls there had been some changes too. Few schools now insisted on the gym slip, mostly the uniform was very similar to that worn by boys, with the exception of trousers, which were definitely not to be adopted by girls who wore instead a pleated skirt, which had to be of a certain length. It was not unusual for girls to be inspected for skirt length – they would have to kneel down, and the hem of their skirt could not be more

than a specified height from the ground.

As the decade wore on several schools tried to become more 'with it' by having new uniforms designed, especially for the girls. Pinafore dresses or tunics were offered as alternatives, and worn over open-necked blouses or a polo-necked jumper or blouse. Skirt lengths were allowed to rise, and tights could be worn. Meanwhile for the boys there might be a relaxation of the rule governing the

Right August 1969 – many schools made drastic changes in their uniforms in the mid to late sixties to try to keep up with changing fashions. Of course with fashion changing so quickly, the idea was doomed to failure.

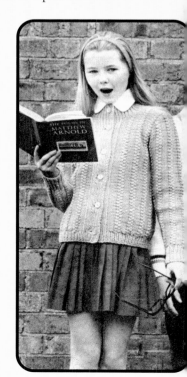

colour of socks, or the need to wear differently coloured shirts in summer and winter! School ties, especially, were a bone of contention, as changing fashions demanded that ties be worn first as slim as possible, then as wide as possible. The more rebellious pupils tried to have their school ties altered to follow the fashion.

Some schools, especially primaries, gave up on school uniform altogether, but most continued to fight a dogged battle with ever-more reluctant pupils to maintain a standard of dress which had largely disappeared from the outside world.

Outside school, children's clothes were as fashionable as most could afford, or as far as

Below Mother and daughter in virtually the same outfits, crocheted mini-dress, white lacy tights and flat shoes. March 1969.

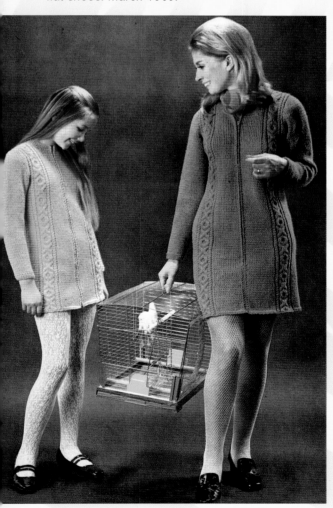

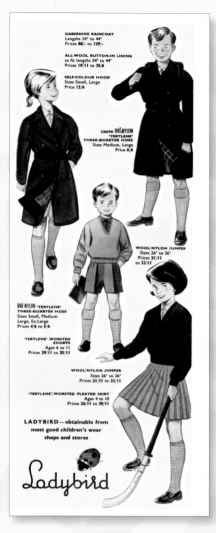

LADYBIRD—obtainable from most good children's wear shops and stores

Ladybird

Left School uniform, August 1961, it's somewhat amazing that over half a century later such outfits are still common.

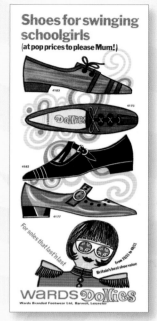

Shoes for swinging schoolgirls (at pop prices to please Mum!)

WARDS Dollies

Wards Branded Footwear Ltd, Barwell, Leicester

Above Advert for girl's shoes, the ad itself being perhaps more remarkable than the shoes - September 1967.

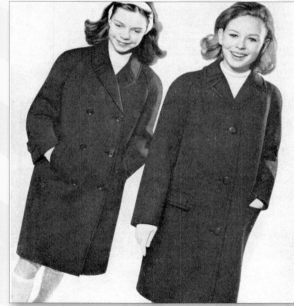

Top of their class

Full marks to these two dannimacs. Hard at work every day, they still manage to look fresh at the end of term. Clever young coats.

Left: the regulation coat. Belted or not. Hood optional (an inside clip in the coat keeps it safe when not in use). From 83/9d.

Right: the classic. Raglan sleeves. Flap pockets. Foam-backed (never creases, never bags). £6.19.6.

BOTH IN GOOD-WEARING GABERDINE

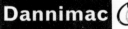**Dannimac**

their parents would let them get away with. There were, of course, still a few who, by choice or more often by parental insistence, would wear their school uniform as their best clothes.

Above Children's raincoats, September 1964.

TEENAGERS

The 1950s saw the emergence of a new type of human individual – the teenager. Previously children had, almost magically, emerged as young adults at about the age of fourteen when most left school, wearing pretty much the same type of clothes as their fathers and mothers did.

Below A teenager in January 1960, dressed in an outfit similar to that worn by his father. Soon the roles would be reversed.

Then, with the start of the post-war consumer boom, teenagers had emerged in the USA, complete with their own fashions, music and even language, and they were rapidly copied by Britain. By then the income of teenagers was 50 per cent higher than it had been pre-war, and it would continue to rise. By the mid-1960s the average teenager was earning £12 to £15 a week. Many teenagers lived away from their family, but the majority still lived at home, so after paying Mum their 'keep', most of their income was disposable, and many would spend up to half of their wages on clothes.

The predominant teenage fashions of the 1950s had been inspired by US rock and roll culture, motorcycle gangs and the Teddy Boys. But for many in the new generation the fashion focus moved from the United States to the continent, in particular France and Italy. Sharp, slim-cut Italian suits were the latest in styling, the motorbike was deposed by Italian motor scooters, while the DA hairstyle was replaced by the French crop.

These forward-looking teenagers became known as 'Mods', short for Modernist, which reflected a passion for the modern jazz of Dave Brubeck and Charlie Mingus as

Right 1961. The baggy sweaters, tapered, striped slacks and hairstyles are still very fifties inspired.

opposed to New Orleans Trad (traditional) jazz. They also listened to black US rhythm and blues music and soul singers.

At the same time, there was a sizeable group who stuck with the old ways, preferring leather jackets, heavily Brylcreemed hair, motorcycles and rock and roll music. This group became known as the

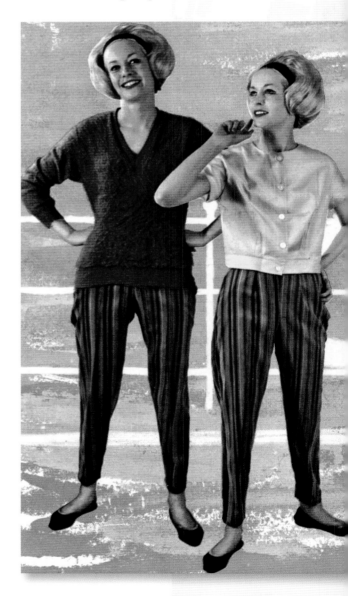

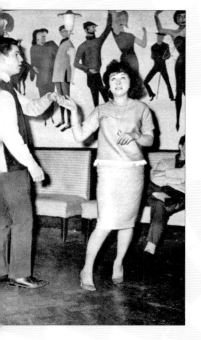

Left *Teenagers at a dance, 1961.*

'Rockers', also from their chosen music, but what really separated the two factions was their choice of clothes. Rockers' outfits were fairly changeless: studded black leather jackets, often with badges – mostly motorcycle related, such as the '59' club, or Nazi regalia – worn over long, usually hand-knitted jumpers for warmth, oil-stained jeans and leather boots. All-in-all, a very practical outfit for riding a motorbike (this kit did not always include a helmet, which was not required by law until 1973). This oil-stained look was viewed with disgust by the impeccably dressed Mods, and led to another derogatory nickname, 'grease' or 'greasers'.

On occasions when a smarter look was required, Rockers might revert to Teddy Boy style, with full drape jackets or at least a long jacket, drainpipe trousers, shoelace tie, and brothel creeper shoes, winklepickers or perhaps cowboy boots worn with the trousers over the top.

The Mods, on the other hand, cared little for practicality. For them, looking sharp was the whole point of clothes, and what mattered most was looking fashionable. For those with lots of disposable income this could be easily achieved; for most with a weekly budget of £5–£10, however, this meant careful shopping around. It helped that fashionable clothes had now become far cheaper, with boutiques offering their wares at very reasonable prices. But the downside of this was that fashions began to change at

an alarming rate. What was 'in' could become laughably 'out' within a few weeks.

There were exceptions. For Mod boys, straight-legged jeans – and that meant Levis – were almost always acceptable, although the length of turn-up, or the absence thereof, signified the wearer's fashionability. Fred Perry polo shirts were another perennial, as were desert boots or Hush Puppies. This made being a Mod expensive. It wasn't just the style that was important, the label had to be right too: sought-after brands included Levis, Fred Perry, Hush Puppies, Pringle pullovers, Crombie overcoats, Ben Sherman shirts and Sta-Prest trousers.

Mod girls tended to wear styles that were soon taken up by older women: miniskirts, bright colours, Op-Art designs, trouser suits, all sprang out of Mod fashions. With good money to be made, shops emerged to cater to the Mods, and between 1962 and 1965 London's Carnaby Street became a focal point for them.

Another Mod trademark was the parka. The **Observer** in March 1967 reported that *'about four years ago, the Mods on their scooters began to feel the winter. The odd rabbit tail was not enough, and they had to look around for warm, cheap clobber. Army surplus supplies were a natural source: parachute jackets, parkas and camouflage trousers filled their immediate needs and a whole new hunting-ground was laid bare.'*

The parka became the thing to wear on a scooter, especially in cold weather, although a suede overcoat, often with a leather collar,

Top *Trouser suit by Hilary Floydd, price 9 gns. Worn with a 'butcher boy' cap. 1968.*
Above *From 'Boyfriend', another very pink party outfit from 1968.*

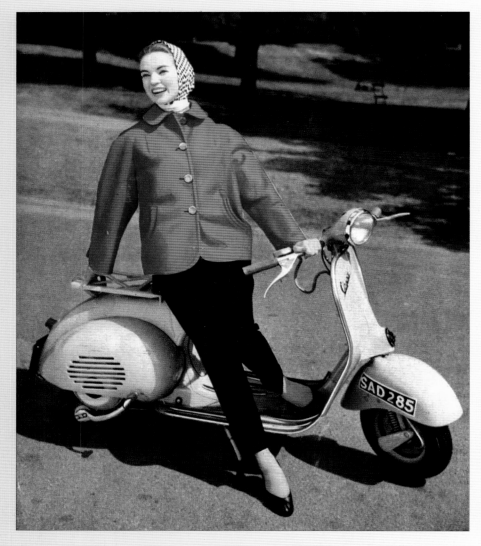

Above *The Vespa motor scooter April 1960. These and Lambrettas would become the hallmarks of the Mods, usually festooned with crash bars and headlamps.*

Right *The shift dress, a perennial favourite, this one from 1968.*

jackets and long, double-vented, three-button jackets with narrow lapels and flap pockets, preferably in 'two-tone' or 'tonic' mohair.

The **Daily Mail** even ran a series entitled 'How to Look Mod in 1963'. In August that year the television music programme **Ready, Steady, Go!** began broadcasting, at 6.06pm on Fridays. The programme, hosted by Keith Fordyce and the 'Queen of the Mods' Cathy McGowan, became a showcase for Mod fashions and music. But the tolerance of the establishment was tested when Mods and Rockers clashed violently on the Easter Bank Holiday weekend of 1964. Large numbers of both groups descending on Clacton-on-Sea, where fights broke out along the seafront. This was followed at Whitsun by similar scenes in Margate and Brighton, and photographs and film of the fighting filled the media.

In the following year, 1965, a schism developed between the 'peacock' or 'smooth' Mods, and the 'hard' or 'gang' Mods (also known as 'lemonheads' or 'peanuts' because of their close-cropped hairstyles). The split came about because one group (the peacock Mods) wanted to move on and become involved in the 'peacock' revolution, in which male fashions became more colourful, flamboyant and, to traditional eyes, effeminate. Prime examples of the peacock style were the Rolling Stones.

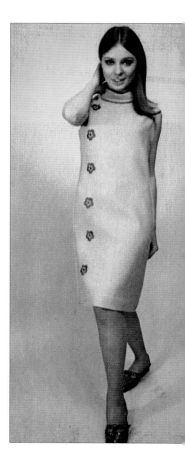

was also acceptable. Parkas were decorated with hand-painted lettering or graphic designs – in 1965 the red, white and blue RAF roundel was widely used as an Op Art-influenced design, and it became a Mod standard. Other badges and military insignia were sewn on to give the wearer a bit of individuality. The parka was often accompanied by a hat, one of the main requirements of which was that it stayed on while riding on a scooter. These included 'pork pie' hats, known as 'blue beat' hats from the popular West Indian music of that name, or shapeless felt hats often covered with badges, Cossack-style fur hats and, of course, crash helmets.

Other Mod fashions included polo or turtleneck sweaters, white trousers, safari

Meanwhile the hard Mods wanted to keep their cropped hair, Sta-Prest trousers, braces, boots and Ben Sherman shirts. Many of the peacock Mods would later become hippies, while the hard Mods became known as skinheads, a style which reached its zenith in 1969.

Having originated in San Francisco, in 1965 hippy culture began to appear in Britain. Hippies were a fusion of several groups: beatniks, folkies, surfers and psychedelics. They were, on the whole, teenagers who had become politicised by the US Civil Rights movement and the Anti-Vietnam War demonstrations, and to this mix were added green politics and anti-consumerism. The movement received the ultimate seal of approval in 1967 when The Beatles went to India to find enlightenment and returned wearing hippy styles: Afghan coats, caftans, cheesecloth shirts and sandals.

The hippies' rejection of the consumer society affected their fashions. The latest high street styles were spurned in favour of second-hand or old clothes that were patched and embroidered, ethnic clothes inspired by Indian or Native American styles, or hand-made clothes like those worn by the early settlers of the American west.

Hippy styles included plain or patterned sheepskin-lined Afghan jackets, waistcoats or full-length coats worn by both sexes, and headbands, often beaded in Native American style. These were worn with embroidered cheesecloth shirts and blouses, or T-shirts, often with jeans, sometimes jean jackets,

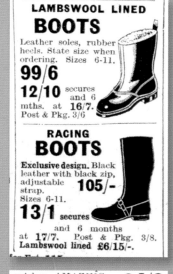

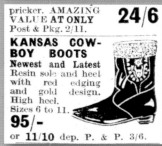

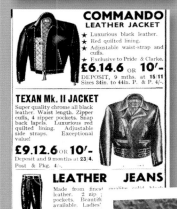

both of which were best faded, ripped and patched, with badge-style embroidered patches typically featuring the CND symbol, slogans such as 'Make Love Not War' or psychedelic artwork. Some girls wore floor-length kaftans. The outfit was completed by long, Native American-style buckskin boots, cowboy boots, plimsolls, sandals or even bare feet, along with beads – 'love beads' as they were called – or a small 'love' bell on a leather thong, beaded bracelets, and rings of every description.

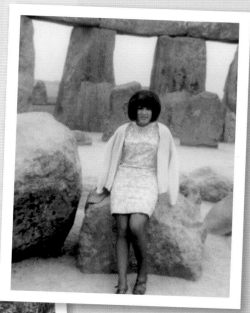

Left, top *Rockers' boots October 1964. Alternatives were army-style boots.*

Mid-left *Another popular rocker boot, the cowboy boot.*

Lower left *Typical rockers' leathers from 1964, the studs and badges would be added by the wearers.*

Above *A very mod hairstyle from the mid-sixties.*

Left *Mods in the late sixties. He still has the mod crop hairstyle, but the long sideburns and moustache are very new. She still wears a mini, and a skinny-rib style jumper, but with Scholl sandals.*

UNISEX

Traditionally men were men and women were women, and their clothes were very different. However, the jumper was one area where there was some overlap, and it became a rather sweet token for young couples to indicate that they were an 'item' by sporting matching hand-knitted pullovers.

A woman wearing a man's shirt as a sort of overall or nightshirt had long been seen as sexy, especially if she were a curvy model in a shirt several sizes too big for her, which had the effect of emphasising her femininity. In 1962 shirt manufacturers took up this idea; **Woman's Mirror** reported in March that *'Like model Sheila Reeve, to get ahead you've got to get a shirt…Sheila decided to try her luck at modelling. It was tough going, until she was chosen to model a man's shirt in an advertisement which is now causing a sensation all over Britain. In the poster Sheila appears to be wearing nothing but a plain white shirt. The caption reads: "It Looks Even Better On A Man."*

'Often it is men's wear she models. That helpless, appealing air of hers makes males rush to photograph her in rugged T-shirts, sweaters and trilby hats. The manufacturers have cottoned on to the idea that there's something fetching about the Girl-In-The-Shirt Look. They're making shirts galore for women…to sleep in, for the beach, or to wear at home as cover-up overalls.'

The French designer Ted Lapidus made the look acceptable, when in his first couture show in 1963 he concentrated on boy/girl fashion mixes, using androgynous models. Reviews spoke of his 'unisex' clothes and the word stuck.

The **Boyfriend Annual** in 1964 reported that *'Gone are the days when women hurried past the dull and dismal clothes stores for men. Now the gay, modern and bright outfits on show make any girl stop and envy the boys their fashions – and often buy them. Shirts, jerkins – yes, and even ties – not to mention hats, are being stolen from the opposite sex as soon as they appear. In fact, today's trend is to match the clothes with the steady boyfriend – and how the heads turn when a good-looking couple stroll hand-in-hand dressed in the same attractive outfits.*

'John Stephen's, the most popular for up-to-date wear for young moderns, are producing more and more casuals that look equally great on your boyfriend and you. Shirts – the most popular item of all stolen from the boys. Most popular of all – the faded denims for the brightest mod!'

Rave magazine in May 1965 declared that *'What should come in VERY big this summer are "Donovan" suits for girls-specially in navy-blue, "faded" denim. To go with them: a big, leather, hipster belt. Shirt can be any bright gingham. Check, preferably. AND, of course, a Donovan cap. Donovan gear is also bang In for boys, too.'*

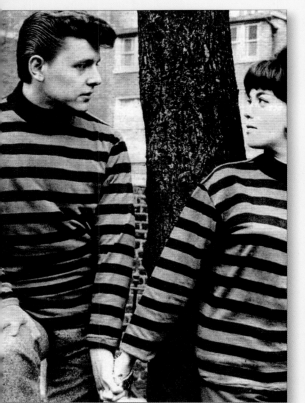

Above *Unisex tops from 1964.*

Opposite page *The matching sweater. The fashion for couples to wear the same patterned sweaters (usually knitted by the girl), was the first emanation of the unisex look, these from 1964.*

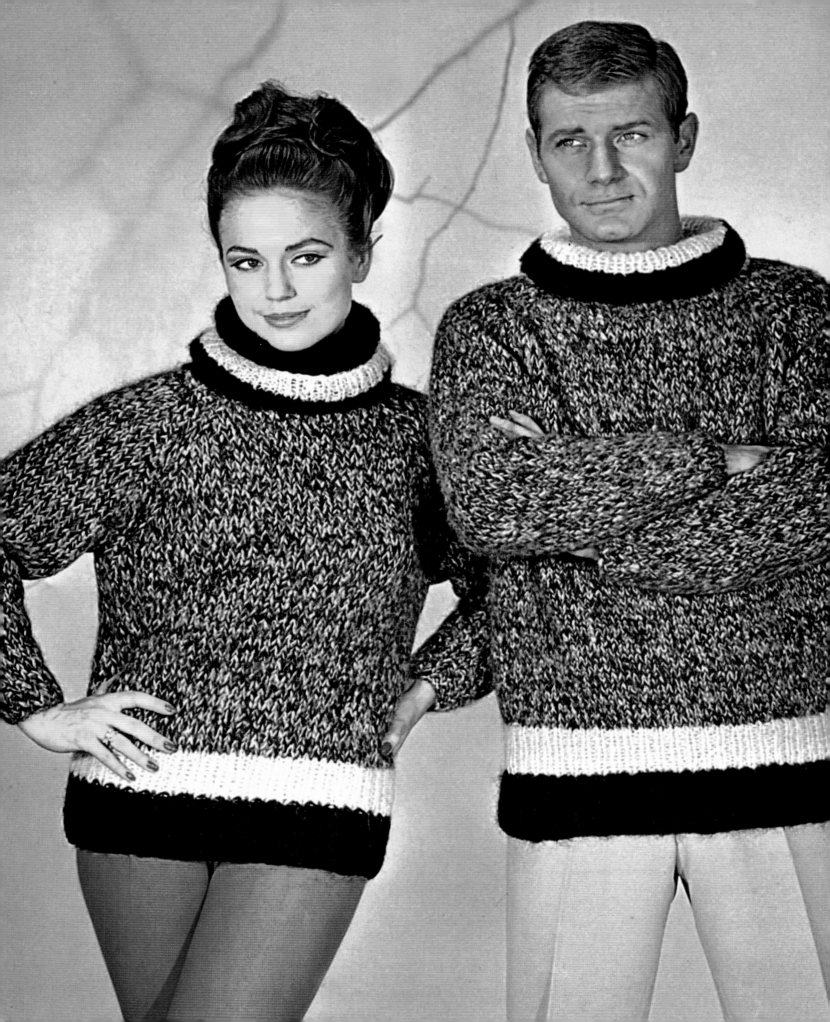

Opposite page, top
Men's shirts had always looked better on women, now men's styles were used for women's blouses, while men's tailoring was used for women's suits and even trousers. October 1963.

Above Donovan, in classic denims and what became known as the Donovan cap. The style was widely copied by both boys and girls, especially the cap. May 1965.

That year's **Boyfriend Annual** declared that *'Where the boys are is where the girls want to be. And the best way of getting there is by wearing the clothes the boys go for. Pretty, pretty styles are okay for girls who like to think they are dolls. But to many a male you can look just as good or even more appealing swathed in leather or slopping around in a pullover three sizes too big. Tough, mannish garments on the "frail" feminine form bring out the tenderness in the he-man, you know. It's true that few boys can resist a pretty girl wearing a waisted frothy dress, but there is something distinctly sexy about the more tom-boyish fashions!'*

The theme, once again, was that it was fine for a girl to wear a man's clothes. Denim was the greatest unisex fashion of all. Jeans started it all off, worn with a shirt, even a denim shirt, a denim waistcoat and jacket. All these were sold equally to both sexes. This was reflected in trouser styles, which were generally based on similar lines, with many women preferring the cut of men's trousers, especially the flat hip fitting. One problem was that, in order to get the right hip size, the waistline would usually be too large, but the introduction of 'hipsters' solved that.

Boyfriend continued: *'Even today's top pop singers like to match the casuals. Below you can see Billie Davis with Neil Christian in cotton-striped sweaters with polo-necks. These sell for about 35s., and come in blue, brown or red with black stripes – and they're chart-toppers if we ever saw any. Ideal for a motor-bike ride, walking or simply shopping. Cool and charming, and if yours gets dirty – why not borrow your brother's? The main article that girls have "pinched" this summer has been the denim shirt. Faded blue has been the most popular and these sell for around 39s. This particular one has two buttons at the pocket and cuffs, and features a line of cotton stitching circling the collar and down from the top button. Fabulous with slacks, very "tourist" with white pleated skirts, these shirts are tops for colours and versatility.*

One thing the boys thought was pretty safe was the waistcoat – but they should have been more careful about showing them off. Boys may look smart in theirs, but have you seen a girl wearing one on top of a silk, long-sleeved shirt blouse? Or with a polo-necked sweater? Absolutely stunning. These waistcoats in French cord come in pillarbox red and black. They may sound a little pricey at 4 guineas, but they certainly won't be pushed into a wardrobe and forgotten. With obvious choice of slacks, or with pleated or straight skirt, they just make the outfit – adding the extra touch to brighten up your WHOLE wardrobe.

'The jerkin looks wonderful with bright shirt blouse and straight skirt. The jerkin costs about 4 guineas, and matching tweed slacks are about 99s.

'Of course, there are many more articles we haven't mentioned – like the cute hats that are just made for girls. Give me a bowler on a girl, any time. And how about knotting his slim-line tie beneath your peter-pan collared blouse? You'll find it adds a lot more to your casual outfit than a string of beads would.'

Vanity Fair, in January 1966, continued the theme, *'…wear anything tattersall check, whether it be dress, suit, skirt, coat, or even a man's shirt. The size of the check doesn't matter, large or small, it's 1966 if it's tattersall. Make blouses, shirts or sweaters look more chic by adding a cravat stolen from men.'*

The fashion for wearing Edwardian-style military jackets continued this theme of girls wearing men's clothes, but genuinely unisex

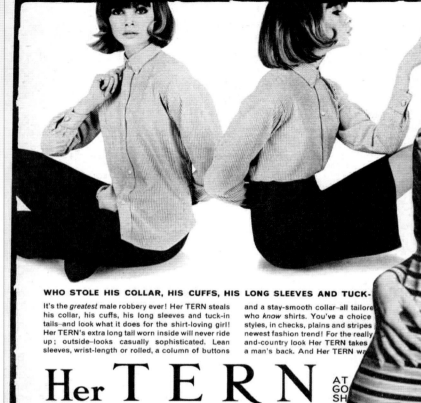

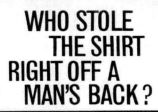

WHO STOLE THE SHIRT RIGHT OFF A MAN'S BACK?

WHO STOLE HIS COLLAR, HIS CUFFS, HIS LONG SLEEVES AND TUCK-

It's the *greatest* male robbery ever! Her TERN steals his collar, his cuffs, his long sleeves and tuck-in tails—and look what it does for the shirt-loving girl! Her TERN's extra long tail worn inside will never ride up; outside–looks casually sophisticated. Lean sleeves, wrist-length or rolled, a column of buttons

and a stay-smooth collar–all tailore who *know* shirts. You've a choice styles, in checks, plains and stripes newest fashion trend! For the really and-country look Her TERN takes a man's back. And Her TERN wa

Her T E R N AT GO SH

For Her TERN leaflet and list of stockists write to:– Londonpride Ltd. (Her TERN Division), 66

fashions also emerged. The 'skinny rib sweater' was one, as were hipster trousers, and fashion pundits predicted that in the future both sexes would wear the same clothes, as was happening in China with the Mao jacket and Red Guard cap. Yet this idea came crashing down in flames as the fashion excesses of 1967–8 began to emerge.

The pendulum had swung the other way; unisex designs were now often based more on women's clothes. Far too often the results looked great on the woman, but nothing short of laughable on the man. Most men, even of the younger generation, soon decided that they would not be seen dead in such outfits, and while denim unisex would continue for many years, other designs, such as unisex cat suits, had a very limited market.

Above Unisex suits, May 1967. The only trouble was that, even at the time, the general opinion was that such suits looked great on the women, but a bit silly on the men.

ACCESSORIES

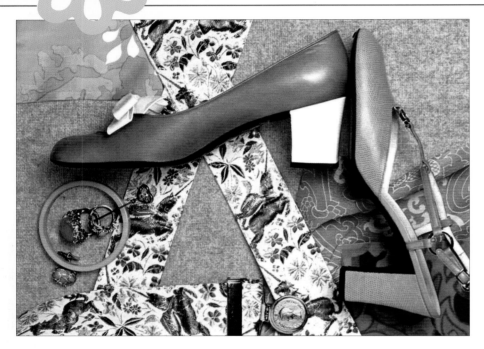

Above *In an era of rapidly changing fashions, accessories; hats, gloves, scarves, belts, etc., could update an outdated costume.*

Right *On the left, the old accessories; white gloves and a matching hat, on the right, the new; co-ordinated beret and bangles.*

Accessories were an important part of any outfit. **Woman** magazine in November 1963 stated that *'As sauces are to cooking so accessories are to clothes. Good ones add spice and flavour that lift an outfit from hum-drum to hot fashion. Bad ones can be dull or over-rich, spoil the whole effect. Key to success, in both cases, is simply getting the mixture right.'*

Woman's Realm in April 1962 opined that *'Dress sense has nothing at all to do with money, and very little to do with the size of your wardrobe. Many of the best-dressed women you meet manage on a tight budget and have extremely few clothes. They choose dateless styles and buy one or two good things each year rather than a lot of cheap ones. And for colour, sparkle and variety they rely on accessories and use these to dress up each outfit and make it look a little bit different for every occasion.'*

In October 1961 **Housewife** told its readers that *'Fabrics, colours and accessories all play an important part in making the finished picture a perfect one, and they should each be chosen with the greatest care and imagination.'*

In the early 1960s dressing stuck to a formula: there were the right things to wear together, and there were the wrong things, and the fashionable woman knew the difference. This awareness was graduated by various subtle nuances, depending on the season, the fashion and your colouring. This advice comes from **Woman's Weekly** in June 1961: *'Would you advise my daughter and myself on what colour accessories to wear with our new Summer suits? Mine is beige linen, with a straight skirt and boxy jacket; I have auburn hair turning grey and blue eyes. My daughter's suit is a muted mid-blue with a pleated skirt and she has dark hair and eyes.'*

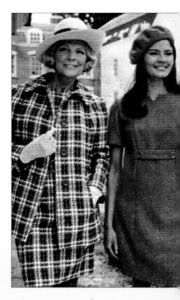

The complexity of the answer speaks volumes about the rules: *'I think that a coffee cream shade would be a good choice for your shoes, bag and gloves; the shoes and bag would look nice in suede, with nylon Simplex for the gloves. Your hat could be a muted turquoise, slate blue, or soft cedar green; I think a toque or small turn-back brim would be flattering.*

'Your daughter could not do better than choose a straw sailor hat – they are perfect on a young face – white would be best with white cotton gloves. Her shoes and bag could be navy leather. Alternatively, she could have light beige for her shoes, bag and gloves with a paler shade of the same blue for her boater.'

In October 1963 the magazine was telling its readers that 'Fashion-conscious women will be on the lookout for bags and shoes that go together this season.' Yet by now the seismic changes that would affect fashion in the 1960s were well underway. Such well-defined rules would be swept away, and replaced simply by the rule that there were no rules – up to a point! Colour prevailed, Perspex jewellery took the place of diamonds, plastic replaced leather, yet certain rules still applied. They were generally tips and tricks to help you minimise, or maximise, your height, weight, hips, chest size etc., and they also related to the accessories you chose. **Woman** magazine gave the following advice in July 1965 to readers who were 'Large – Buy accessories that minimise – chunky jewellery your size can take; narrow bags that cut your width; broad-brimmed hats that balance hips; new lace-up look for shoes.

'Small – Choose accessories scaled to size – be the height of fashion with a neat chain-handled shoulder-bag merged into the background of your clothes; bowed, flowered or spotted shoes; cute crochet beret or flowered snood.

'Tall – Don't be afraid to accessorise, you're the girl who can wear (and get away with) big, big sunglasses; huge portmanteaux or carpet bags; fancy vamp shoes and those gorgeous hats My Fair Lady inspired.'

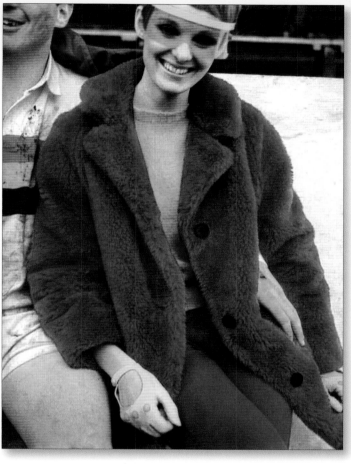

Left The latest accessories in 1966, cut-away gloves (later, driving gloves), space age visor, and coloured fun fur.

One of the biggest changes related to the actual pace at which fashions changed. Clothes became cheaper as small boutiques sprang up, but the latest crazes came and went with amazing rapidity. However, the advice of **Woman's Realm** in 1962 still rang true; on a limited budget, accessories could work wonders on a restricted wardrobe. Thus the importance of accessories increased, and the profiles of their designers were raised at the same time. Clothes designers such as Cardin and Quant had long been fêted, and had on occasions moved into designing accessories, but now accessory designers began to receive similar acclamation. 'Teasie-Weasy' Raymond and Vidal Sassoon became celebrity hairdressers, Charles Jourdan and Roger Vivier noted shoe designers (both for Christian Dior), James Wedge was applauded for jewellery and millinery, and Oliver Goldsmith for spectacles.

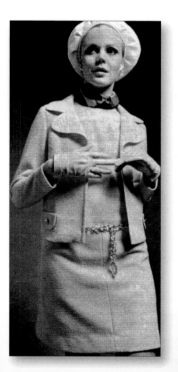

Above Gloves were still a popular accessory, but you were no longer restricted to white cotton or lace – these from January 1969.

SHOES

When the 1960s began, most people were still wearing shoes that would not have looked out of place in the 1940s. As with the rest of fashion, this was about to change. The emphasis soon would be on the casual, with the humble plimsoll undergoing radical changes that saw it take on colour and styling to develop into the sneaker, which in turn later morphed into the trainer.

Below Sneekers casuals, April 1965, one of the missing links between the plimsol and the trainer.

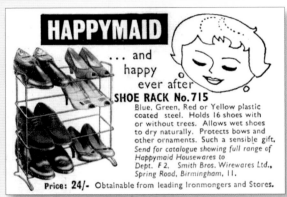

Other long-ignored items of footwear became newly popular, including the elastic-sided boot, Cuban heels, the suede desert boot, and most of all the long boot, soon to be renamed the 'kinky' boot. This was mainly for women, although men too would take to boot-wearing.

Men

The fashion for an overall slim line extended to men's shoes in the form of the pointed, long-toed winklepicker, most fashionably in a half-length elastic-sided Chelsea boot. This style had previously been much favoured by army officers as the plain front formed an uninterrupted line under trousers devoid of turn-ups.

Men Only in October 1961 reported that *'There is a pronounced trend to softer, lighter shoes for town and country wear. The accent is more and more on extra flexibility and soft leathers which are easy to clean. Black as a colour stays as stable as a rock in its sales, but for the autumn browns are expected to be popular. They will be darker browns like the latest shades in suitings. Cherrywood, tobacco, acorn and teak, with the addition of a new dark*

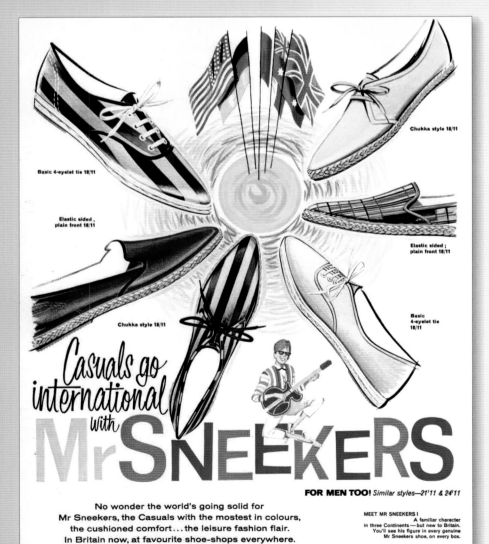

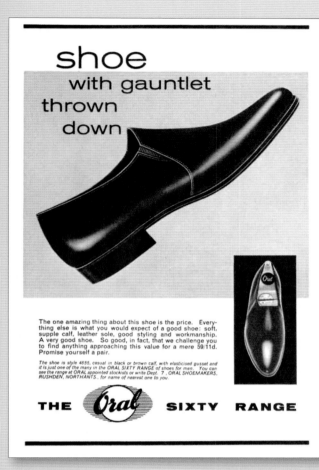

shoe
with gauntlet
thrown
down

The one amazing thing about this shoe is the price. Everything else is what you would expect of a good shoe: soft, supple calf, leather sole, good styling and workmanship. A very good shoe. So good, in fact, that we challenge you to find anything approaching this value for a mere 59/11d. Promise yourself a pair.

The shoe is style 4655, casual in black or brown calf, with elasticised gusset and it is just one of the many in the ORAL SIXTY RANGE of shoes for men. You can see the range at ORAL appointed stockists or write Dept. 7 , ORAL SHOEMAKERS, RUSHDEN, NORTHANTS, for name of nearest one to you.

THE *Oral* SIXTY RANGE

boots, often army surplus models, for more manual jobs, with perhaps a pair of brogues for going out, and possibly a suede pair for more casual wear.

In February 1962 **Men Only** predicted that *'for the trend-setter, one pair of summer shoes will incorporate interlacing or mesh. The interlacing may be printed rather than genuinely woven, but it will be seen as fronts or decorations on both men's and women's shoes. New for men this summer will be Chelsea boots with square toes, spade-like duckbill toes, and the matchbox line – a rather sharp, chopped-off, raised square toe.'*

In 1963–4 the popularity of The Beatles and their look encouraged the rapid take-up of these elastic-sided Chelsea boots, but at first with pointed toes and high, Cuban heels which became known as Beatle boots. These were superseded by the square-cut 'chisel' toe.

Hush Puppies had been introduced in 1958 as a rubber-soled suede shoe for 'tired feet'. They were popular with older people,

Left *Men's elastic sided shoe, May 61. These became very popular, as the flat front did not affect the slim-line look created by narrow trousers.*

Below left *Casuals from America, April 1966.*

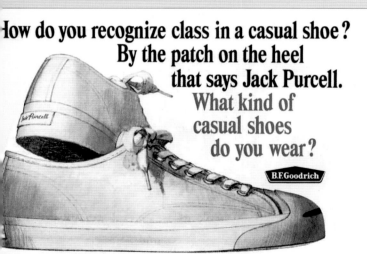

How do you recognize class in a casual shoe?
By the patch on the heel
that says Jack Purcell.
What kind of
casual shoes
do you wear?

B.F.Goodrich

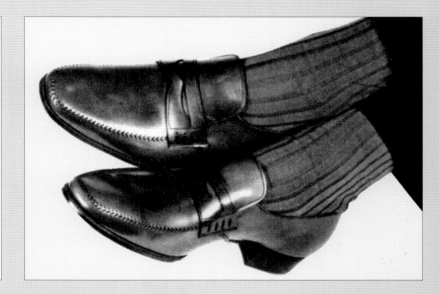

greenish colour called burnt olive, are some of the names to look out for.'

In the early 1960s Cardin had introduced mid-calf length 'Space-Boots' for men in his collection. Most men, however, continued to wear the lace-up shoe in plain black or brown for clerical-type work, or lace-up

but little loved by the younger generation. However, one of the early Mod fashions was for safari jackets, worn with desert boots, a type of a suede half-boot. This then led to Mods adopting the Hush Puppy or other suede casuals, and they would remain a perennial part of Mod fashions.

Above right *June 1968, the chisel toe is still in, now slightly softened, while the elastic-sided boot has become the 'step in'.*

Other styles which caught on in the
second half of the decade were slip-ons.
These, like sneakers, looked right with jeans
– by then almost universally worn by anyone
under thirty.

The advent of the hippies introduced
Native American-style boots with fringed
tops, usually worn with trousers or jeans
tucked into them. Boots were also made of
suede or leather patchwork. In a further nod
to the Native American
influence, moccasins,
sometimes with beadwork,
were popular, as were sandals.
Some brave souls even went
barefoot.

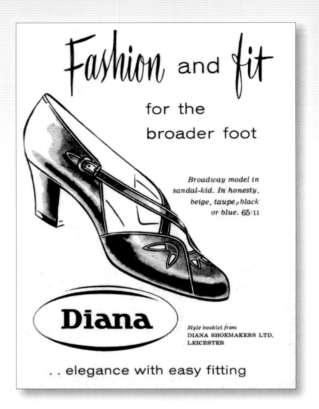

Fashion and fit
for the
broader foot

*Broadway model in
sandal-kid. In honesty,
beige, taupe, black
or blue. 65/11*

Diana

Style booklet from
DIANA SHOEMAKERS LTD.
LEICESTER

.. elegance with easy fitting

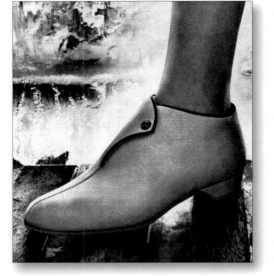

Women

At the start of the decade
women's shoes were still very
similar in style to those of the
1940s and 1950s. Colours were
muted, and heels for daywear
shoes were of medium length
– 2 to 2½ inches – and

thickness. The most common shape was a
low slip-on, with a rounded point to the toe.

For summer wear a similar shape was
common, medium-heeled but with an open
front. This style was termed a sandal, and to
match the brighter clothes worn during the
summer months, they were often far more
brightly coloured.

Evening shoes often had longer, thinner
stiletto heels, and might be more decorated
than day models, manufactured in
combinations of suede and leather, and/or
pierced brogue-style.

Writing in **Woman** magazine in January
1961, Veronica Scott told her readers that
*'Shopping for shoes in 1961 is simple. Toes
stay long and mostly pointed, but there's a
feeling afoot for oval toes, and the squared
point, too.*

*'Textures are mixed with gay, and
glamorous, abandon. Plain and patent
leather…pearlized leather with plush
pigskin…canvas and leather…patent
leather with flannel.*

*'Trims on almost every shoe are neat
little tie-bows used as laces or simply for*

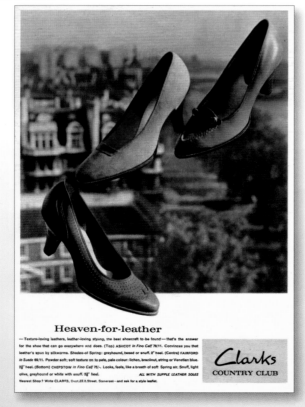

Heaven-for-leather

— Texture-loving leathers, leather-loving styling, the best shoecraft-to-be found—that's the answer
for the shoe that can go everywhere and does. (Top) ASHCOT *in Fino Calf* 79/11. Convinces you that
leather's spun by silkworms. Shades-of-Spring: greyhound, tweed or snuff. 2" heel. (Centre) FAIRFORD
in Suede 69/11. Powder soft; soft texture on to pale, pale colour: lichen, brazilnut, string or Venetian blue.
2¼" heel. (Bottom) CHEPSTOW *in Fino Calf* 75/-. Looks, feels, like a breath of soft Spring air. Snuff, light
olive, greyhound or white with snuff. 2¼" heel.   ALL WITH SUPPLE LEATHER SOLES
Nearest Shop? Write CLARKS, Dept.ZE.9,Street. Somerset—and ask for a style leaflet.

Clarks
COUNTRY CLUB

fun. Tongues or a little punching are the only other decorations. The tailored look is tops.

'Heels? Rushing into top place comes stacked leather, real or simulated. Favourite heights run from 1½ to 2½ in.

'The colour picture shows brown, with chocolate brown first favourite, even for summer sandals. Black comes next in line, with greens and apricot following close behind.'

Lower 'kitten' heels were an alternative to stilettos, while for country wear or casual wear flat-soled shoes, often in suede or calf, were fashionable.

As ever, the cold and wet weather of a British winter caused many women to opt for comfort over fashion, and there were many variations on the lined winter boot.

In 1962 the pattern changed very little. The options were the stout country shoe –

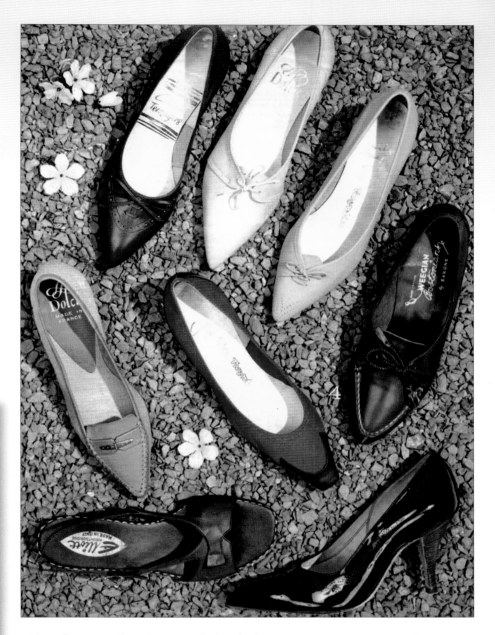

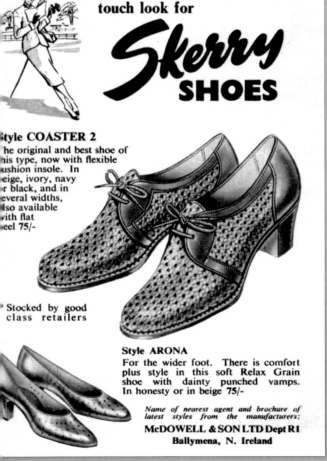

either flat or with a short, wide heel; the town day shoe – usually a court shoe, with a higher thinner heel; the winter boot, or high-sided bootee; and the evening shoe, often with a higher or even stiletto heel. Toes could be found in the whole range of shapes: the rounded point, the point and the newly fashionable chisel.

Modern Woman in September predicted that 'High fashion for your feet, this Autumn, will be the reptiles – crocodile, alligator, lizard, snakeskins like python. They're pretty hardwearing and, for the first time, at prices to suit all pockets.'

Above *An excellent example of the wide range of the shoes, moccasins and sandals, the materials; suede, leather, pigskin, canvas and patent, and the colours which were available in January 1961.*

Left *April 1962, and the top shoes could be from 1942, or even earlier.*

Left Clarks fashion shoes from September 1965.
Far left Boots, October 1964, while short, and even high heels could be seen, the main fashion look in boots was a low heel, or even a flat sole.

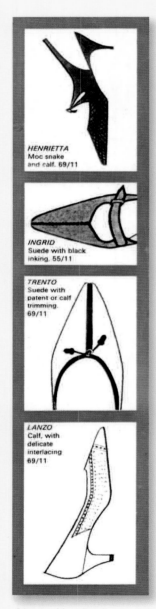

HENRIETTA
Moc snake and calf. 69/11

INGRID
Suede with black inking. 55/11

TRENTO
Suede with patent or calf trimming. 69/11

LANZO
Calf, with delicate interlacing 69/11

Above Norvic shoes, April 1965.
Right October 1963, throughout the middle sixties, flat shoes would be the norm.

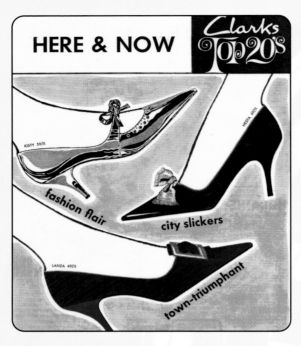

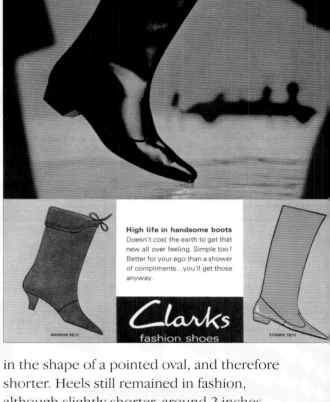

High life in handsome boots
Doesn't cost the earth to get that new all over feeling. Simple too ! Better for your ego than a shower of compliments...you'll get those anyway.

Woman's Realm that April showed its readers how to achieve a *'New look for old shoes – For just a few shillings you can give a new party gloss to shoes which are badly marked. You can give a new lease of life to badly marked, light-coloured court shoes, or change ordinary day shoes into glamorous evening slippers at little cost by spraying them carefully with two or three coats of gold or silver lacquer. This is available, price 4s. 6d. a tin, with aerosol spray from your local chain store. For an extra luxury touch, make a bow or rosette trimming from gold or silver ribbon. Glue this to an ear-ring clip, which you can buy from any handicraft shop, and clip the trimming on to the front of the shoe.'*

In 1963 the rather formidable winklepicker toe became a more muted almond toe; it was still pointed, but now more in the shape of a pointed oval, and therefore shorter. Heels still remained in fashion, although slightly shorter, around 2 inches being the norm for day shoes.

Flat heels were popular for country shoes, but they were also becoming increasingly the vogue among younger women for everyday wear in any situation. Another style which soon took off in a big way was the boot, although at this point most boots still had a high heel, some even stiletto, and were seen as cold or wet weather wear. Here too, however, the flat heel was beginning to appear.

In 1964 the 'Swinging 1960s' were beginning to take hold. Fashionable shoes were still mainly almond-toed, but now in bright colours, or with a buckle front. Buckle-fronted shoes in patent leather were very fashionable; some were made with matching buckles and heels in silver or gold.

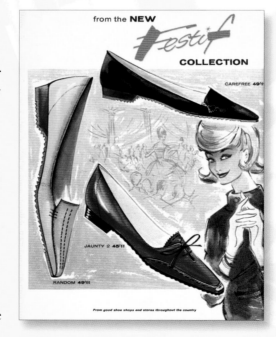

from the NEW *Festif* COLLECTION

The stiletto was still stylish among older women, but the strongly emerging teenage look leaned towards a shorter, thicker heel, or even flat shoes.

Boots were also being worn by the younger set, again with low or flat heels, but as **Modern Woman** told its readers that October: '*…not often above the calf – at the ankle for pant-suits.*' While '*you can wear high heels with trousers (says Chanel), but the trousers must be ankle length and the heels cannot be more than 2in. high.*'

Over the next few years, the dominance of the young look, and its signature fashion, the miniskirt, would dictate the form that footwear would take. Pointed and chiselled toes didn't suit the mini, thin heels also

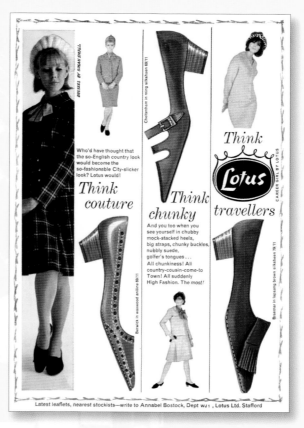

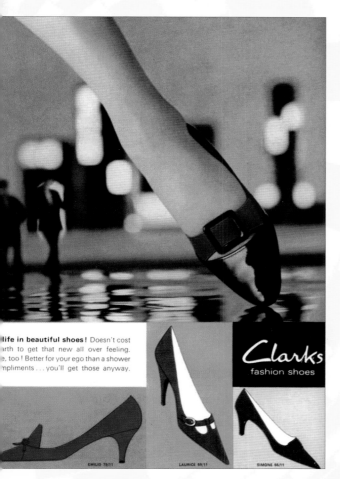

life in beautiful shoes! Doesn't cost arth to get that new all over feeling. e, too! Better for your ego than a shower mpliments … you'll get those anyway.

Clarks fashion shoes

EMILIO 79/11   LAURICE 59/11   SIMONE 55/11

looked wrong, while the added height given by the stiletto was at odds with a younger look. The vibrant, athletic mood suited a shoe that looked as if you could run in it.

Left As the advert points out, the country walking shoe had become the height of fashion by October 1964.

Far left October 1964 – the top shoe, with its bar and large buckle, was particularly fashionable.

Below right A good range of fashionable shoes, October 1964.

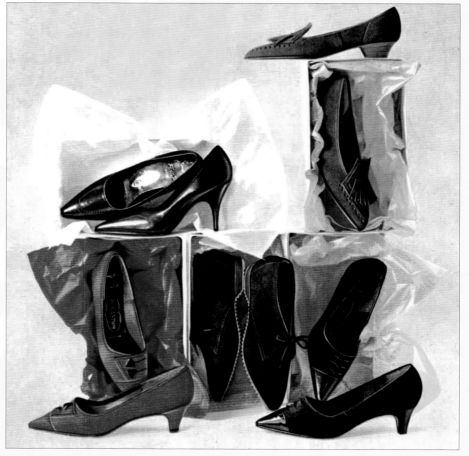

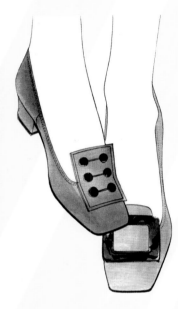

Right *September 1966, the flat suede shoe was a perennial favourite, teaming up very well with the mini skirt.*

Above *Regency-style buckled shoes from 1968.* **Below** *A wide range of brightly-coloured boots from October 1968.*

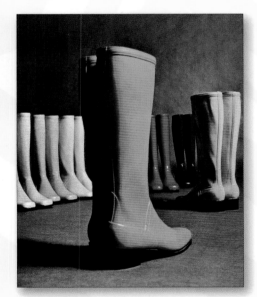

Far right *The latest (1968) thigh-length patent boot with elasticated top, better known as 'kinky boots'.*

Mod boys had originally discovered the Hush Puppy, but in line with the unisex theme prevalent in 1965, girls soon took them up; they were perfect for the fashionable sporty look.

Heels were still in use for evening wear, but they were shorter than usual. **Rave** magazine that May asked its readers *'Who's for 'In' shoes? Get them with small, thick heels. Right now I'm overboard for shoes with big geometric cut-outs. Look for Royal College of Art designs sold by Lotus.'*

Boots were fashionable at any length. As the **Boyfriend Annual** in 1965 stated: *'We all know about leather or imitation leather boots. Ankle length, calf length, knee-high, above the knees and thigh-high. We've all got a pair.'*

As hemlines soared in 1966, so flat boots became very popular; The long-legged mini-style looked great on girls with perfect legs, but for the less fortunate boots offered a way around the problem. As the hemline rose, so did the height of the boots, from mid-calf to knee-length and even thigh-length. These widish, supple boots soon became known as 'kinky boots'; in Paris Courrèges produced white kidskin boots and Saint Laurent thigh-high alligator-skin boots.

The miniskirt's unforgiving focus on the leg could be avoided by the use of trousers, but many turned to exercise as a way of improving the shape and tone of their legs. One variation on this was to wear Dr Scholl sandals.

William Scholl had come across wooden sandals in Germany at the end of the Second World War. He developed the design, adding

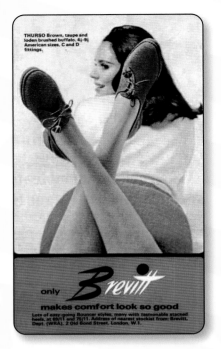

a coloured leather strap, and in 1959 it was launched as the 'Original Exercise Sandal', with the claim that wearing it toned the leg muscles. This sales line, its flat sole and primary-coloured strap were made for the mid 1960s, and they would remain in fashion for many years.

In 1967 boots remained in fashion, while, as an alternative, black or white wet-look leggings were worn with patent or wet-look shoes. For those who could not afford long kid-leather boots, wet-look plastics were perfect for both boots and leggings. Du Pont's 'Corfam', a leather look-alike, was considered the healthiest of the synthetics as it allowed the foot to breathe. In that year Mary Quant produced her first collection of boots: *'In crystal clear plastic over colours that zoom into fashion's orbit, they're boots that shrug off wear and weather marks, come up shining. Five*

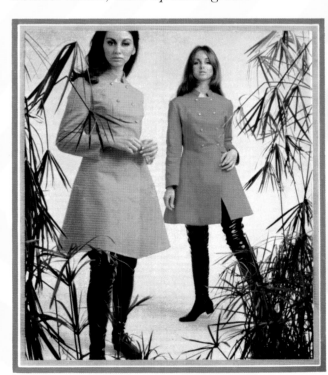

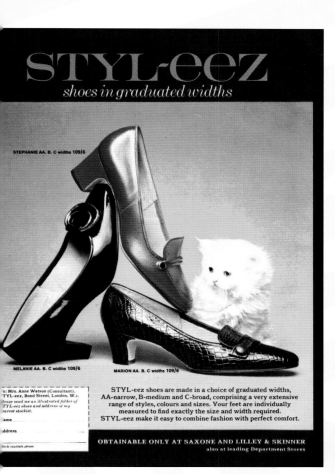

different styles, all with the uncluttered, unmistakable Quant touch, all in a choice of colours.'

Shoes and boots continued to be flat or have low heels; Dior's models wore perspex heels, while Charles Jourdan introduced the doubled-up rounded heel. A retro strand to 1960s fashions produced shoes with the feel of the 1920s, '30s or '40s, with Vivier reviving the 1940s platform shoe. In September 1967 **Woman** magazine informed its readers that *'Shoes are getting roomier and squarer, with chunky fronts and higher, thicker squared-off heels.'*

In 1968 the continued popularity of the miniskirt meant that the polar extremes of boots and Dr Scholl's remained as popular as ever.

Knitted tights, often in white, were popular summer wear, setting of brightly coloured shoes and boots. For the winter tights were usually in dark colours. Shoes

were getting noticeably heavier-looking with broader, thicker heels and round toes. The retro look was still the most fashionable, with the small platform soles which Vivier had introduced the previopus year beginning to appear in high-street shops.

1969 was epitomised by the romantic look, but this was also the time when the 1960s began to lose their way and the styles that would characterise the 1970s emerged. By the autumn of 1969 the platform shoe, which had seen some popularity in 1968, was the

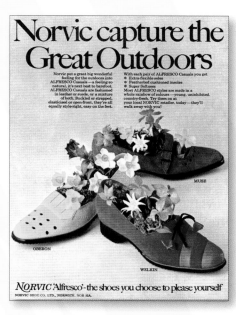

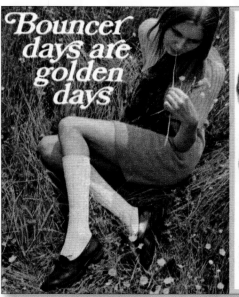

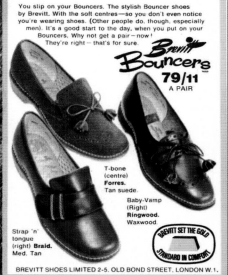

prevailing fashion. **Vogue** explained to its readers: *'Clunk, clunk, sschump, sschump, bump…No more clickety, click, tippy, tap, tap – it's the new sound of soles we're talking about the soles of shoes and sandals are now lifted, thickened, platformed.'*

The romantic fashion looked to Laura Ashley-style country life with shoes that harked back to the sandals worn by children, or to the Biba-style Edwardian look – black stockings worn with black leather or suede, high, lace-up shoes. Another retro style harked back towards the fashions of the 1940s. Look out – here come the 1970s!

Above More child-like shoes, this time from September 1969.

Top left 'Styl-eez shoes in graduated widths' November 1969.

Top right Extremely fashionable chunky suede shoes from April 1968.

Socks, Stockings and Tights

Socks

Men's socks had undergone a revolution in the previous decade with man-made fibres largely replacing wool, resulting in socks which were thin and well-fitting. Shapeless socks which bunched around the ankle were only for old men, and the archaic alternatives, long socks with garters or sock-suspenders, were only seen in comic strips.

Socks came in a huge range of colours, and fashions in socks changed. **Men Only** in October 1961 reported that, *'This autumn men will be putting back the clox-on socks. They will be found on short styles as well as half-hose. Some will be hand-embroidered, others woven-in. These socks can be bought in manmade yarns – nylon, Terylene and mixtures – as well as wool.'*

Long socks were rarely fashionable, and nor were patterns such as Argyle; plain was usually safe, but the colour could be critical. In 1965, for example, white was all the rage, later to be replaced by bright red, blue or yellow.

For the first time since the 1940s women also began to wear socks. The fashionable child-like look was achieved by the wearing of bobby socks, while miniskirts and dresses were complemented by long socks, and sometimes even football socks.

Stockings

Stockings, or nylons as they were universally known, had improved immensely as a result of the use of man-made fabrics. They were still commonly sold with a seam down the back. In the spring of 1960 the fashionable colour in stockings among the young was

black. One reader wrote to **Woman's Realm** that March to say: *'How fashions change. I loathed wearing long black stockings when I was at school. Now my young daughter is begging me for a pair so that she can be in the fashion.' By 1961, Tan-tan Bri-Nylon*

Right The mini proved a problem – stocking tops and suspenders showed – one answer was long socks. October 1966.

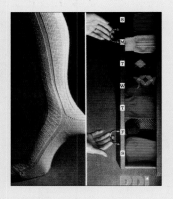

Above April 1962, the 'peacock revolution', whereby men's dress became more flamboyant started in a small way with ties and socks.

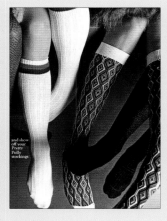

Above Long socks became the rage as minis got shorter. October 1966.

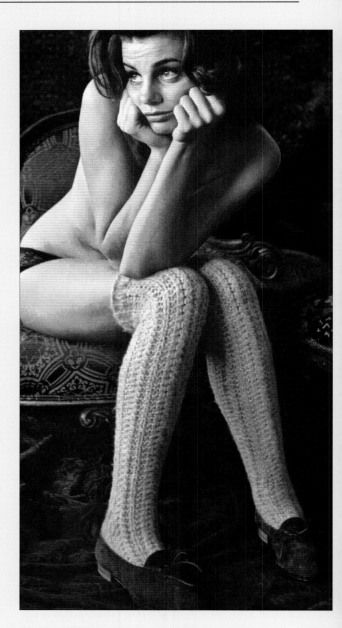

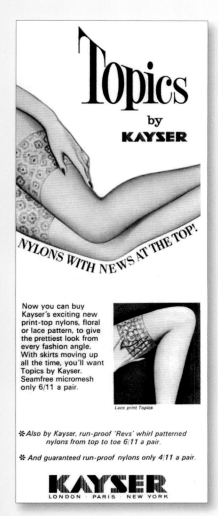

Topics by KAYSER

NYLONS WITH NEWS AT THE TOP!

Now you can buy Kayser's exciting new print-top nylons, floral or lace pattern, to give the prettiest look from every fashion angle. With skirts moving up all the time, you'll want Topics by Kayser. Seamfree micromesh only 6/11 a pair.

Lace print Topics

❊ *Also by Kayser, run-proof 'Revs' whirl patterned nylons from top to toe 6/11 a pair.*

❊ *And guaranteed run-proof nylons only 4/11 a pair.*

KAYSER
LONDON · PARIS · NEW YORK

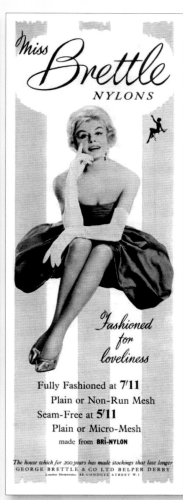

Miss **Brettle** NYLONS

Fashioned for loveliness

Fully Fashioned at **7/11**
Plain or Non-Run Mesh
Seam-Free at **5/11**
Plain or Micro-Mesh
made from **BRI-NYLON**

The house which for 200 years has made stockings that last longer
GEORGE BRETTLE & CO LTD BELPER DERBY
London Showrooms: 48 CONDUIT STREET W.1

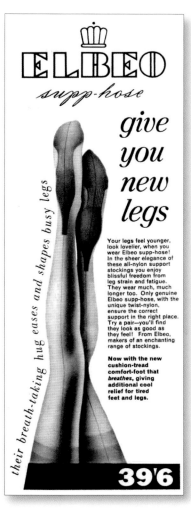

ELBEO *supp-hose*

give you new legs

Your legs feel younger, look lovelier, when you wear Elbeo supp-hose! In the sheer elegance of these all-nylon support stockings you enjoy blissful freedom from leg strain and fatigue. They wear much, much longer too. Only genuine Elbeo supp-hose, with the unique twist-nylon, ensure the correct support in the right place. Try a pair—you'll find they look as good as they feel! From Elbeo, makers of an enchanting range of stockings.

Now with the new cushion-tread comfort-foot that *breathes*, giving additional cool relief for tired feet and legs.

their breath-taking hug eases and shapes busy legs

39'6

Far left Ever-shorter minis meant that stocking-tops were often on show, so why not make a virtue of necessity, April 1966.

Middle left In June 1960 a woman had to make other choices than just the stockings' colours, now there were seamed, or seam-free, but later there would be even more choices.

Left October 1961, most stockings still had seams.

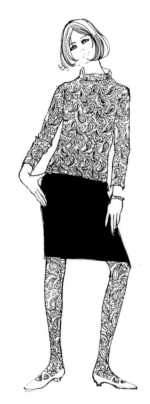

seamless stockings could be bought in a range of colours including mandarin, suntan, bronztone, tortoiseshell, coffee or charcoal, and all for 5s 11d a pair.'

Thicker, knitted stockings became popular. Not only were they warmer in the winter, but with rising hemlines they looked good. **Modern Woman** commented in October 1964: *'The fashionable way to show a smart leg this winter will be to wear patterns; the more riotous the better. Choose large designs for thin legs, and small for plump ones. These warm stockings are in crimped nylon and Terylene, stretched for a good fit. The bold Argyll tartan is made in four colours. Patterned stockings cost from about 12s 11d a pair.'*

By May 1965 **Rave** magazine was telling its readers that *'OUT go weird and wonderful designs. Plain, seamless stockings are In.*

Colours for shoes and stockings: beige or thereabouts.' However, with the fashion pendulum swinging wildly, by that autumn patterns were back in, the more extreme the better, as hemlines rose once again. Most fashionable of all was wearing stockings and blouse to match, preferably in paisley.

The rise in hemlines was all very well for those with perfect legs, but for those who hadn't **Woman** offered a solution in July 1965. *'Slim with stockings that shade to flatter thick ankles or calves, 12s 11d; relieve weary legs with super-strong supporting sheer stretch nylon, 39s 6d. Both by Elbeo, seamed and seamfree.'*

Tights

The ever-rising hemline led inevitably to the shortest of minis, commonly nicknamed the pelmet, meaning that St Trinian's-style

Above Set of matching paisley patterned stockings and sweater in Bri-nylon - £2 9s 11d the set, at Richard Shops, Autumn 1965.

flashes of suspenders were inevitable. One solution was tights or, as they were known, pantyhose. Tights had been used in the entertainment business for years, but it was only in the mid 1950s that Allen Gant developed what were later called 'Panti-Legs', the world's first commercial tights. They went on sale in 1959.

However, not all women liked them. **Woman's Own** in April 1968 outlined the alternatives. *'Here's what's happening if you don't wear tights: If you don't wear tights because you can't get them to fit, here's good news for you. Girdle Hose, made by Kayser, is a pantie girdle with bra-like hooks. It hooks on to extra long stretch stockings with an elastic net top, so there's no ugly gap between stocking top and girdle. You buy the girdle to fit your hips, the stockings to fit your legs. Girdles, 29s 11d, stockings 9s 11d a pair.*

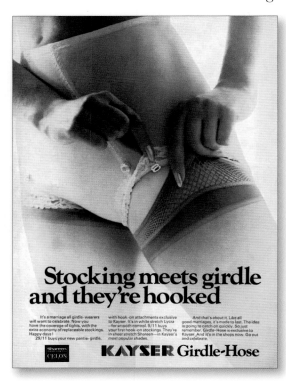

Stocking meets girdle and they're hooked

It's a marriage all girdle-wearers will want to celebrate. Now you have the coverage of tights, with the extra economy of replaceable stockings. Happy days!
29/11 buys your new pantie-girdle,

with hook-on attachments exclusive to Kayser. It's in white stretch Lycra —for smooth control. 9/11 buys your first hook-on stockings. They're in sheer stretch Shareen—in Kayser's most popular shades.

And that's about it. Like all good marriages, it's made to last. The idea is going to catch on quickly. So just remember. Girdle-Hose is exclusive to Kayser. And it's in the shops now. Go out and celebrate.

Shareen
CELON

KAYSER Girdle-Hose

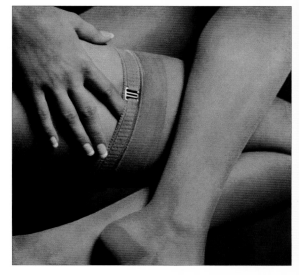

'If you want to steer clear of both hooks and suspenders look out for "Grippernickers" by Lovable. It's a Lycra tricot pantie girdle with a band of Lycra grip elastic in the leg that grips on to the stockings and holds them up. The girdle comes in one size to fit up to a 38-in. hip. The stockings come in three sizes; small, medium and large. A pack of girdle and stockings costs 29s 11d, and you buy it by your own stocking size. The girdle on its own costs 25s 11d, and the stockings cost 4s 11d a pair.

'Alternatively, wear self-support stockings that literally stay up by themselves. No suspenders, no hooks or garters, they are kept up by a band of rubberized elastic that clings to your legs. Charnos "Top Notch" self-supports have a clip so you can adjust the length of the elastic to suit your thighs. They cost 9s 11d a pair. Pretty Polly have four styles in their "Hold Up" range. Ballito are the only people who make textured self supports. Called Sea Witch, they are a lacy design and cost 12s 11d a pair.

While *'…if you still wear stockings: they're getting more sheer but more hard-wearing, flexible and softer to touch. This is due to the development of new yarns like*

Soflons, Shareen and Nystop, which feel softer and have greater powers of recovery. Sounds technical, but it means that when you bend the yarn bends with you and then springs back into shape! Stockings are getting longer, to wear under the mini. Look for Pex "Long Legs" and Wolsey "Highlight". Textures are more exciting, like Bear Brand's "Scrumble" which has a boucle effect. Sales of support stockings – which are getting more sheer everyday – are booming as women spend more time on their feet. And finally, the 30's look has hit stockings. Ann Ford has designed a Bonnie & Clyde leg look for Bear Brand. Fully fashioned, it has a Cuban heel and a thick black seam! Seams? Yes, looking into our crystal ball, we believe they'll be making a big leg fashion come-back very soon.'

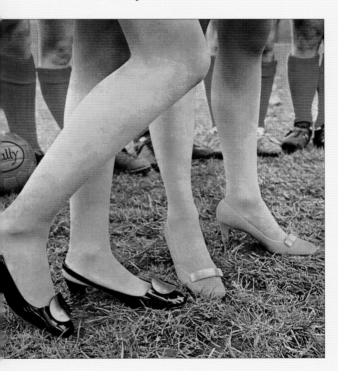

In September 1967, **Woman** magazine advised that 'stockings, tights should tone with shoes, in textures ranging from cobweb crochet, to thick country cousin "handknits". Most sought-after shades of the season: bitter chocolate, navy.'

Woman's Own in April 1968 reported that 'tights have taken over a quarter of all hosiery sales. Prices: They are still relatively high in comparison with stockings, though Woolworth prices now start at 6s 11d, Marks and Spencer at 7s 11d. Average price, however, is now about 10s 11d.

'Sizing. The old problems remain, though manufacturers to whom we put your constant complaints about badly-fitting tights insist that half the battle is buying the right size. And how do you know which is the right size? They're generally graded small (8 1/2–9 stocking size), medium (9 1/2–10) and large (10 1/2–11). Among the exceptions are Wolsey, who size theirs by height (Petite, Average, Tall and Extra Tall), and Woolworth who grade one of their tights range by both stocking size and height.

'Tights to help you make the change over: If you still want to wear a girdle that has non-detachable suspenders underneath, Wolsey Super-Tights have a band of fabric knitted in at stocking top level to which you can fix and tuck away your suspenders. They cost 14s 11d a pair. If you want tights with tummy control, look for Charnos "Hold Me Tights". These are 20 denier crepe micro mesh tights with a built in crepe and Lycra pantie girdle. Price 16s 11d. "Legs by Read" are two stockings hooked together to form tights. When one leg ladders, you replace it with another. A very good budget buy, it costs 10s 11d for a pack of three stockings.'

One innovation which did not catch on – "Sleekers" – was reported by **Honey** magazine in January 1968. 'Specially hardwearing tights with the feet dipped and moulded in crystal-clear plastic, you just pop the lot in your weekly wash. You can buy Sleekers in white, black, camel, khaki, grey, and yellow, in short, medium and long lengths. and shoe sizes 3–7 (with half sizes). Price of this answer to a maiden's prayer: 39s 11d by Mary Quant.'

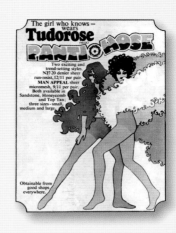

Above The ultimate answer to the mini, tights, or as they were then called – pantyhose, April 1968.

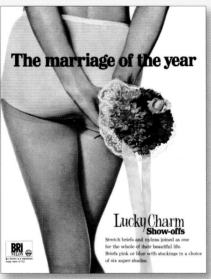

Above Combination pants and nylons, October 1968.

Far left Very orange tights, April 1969.

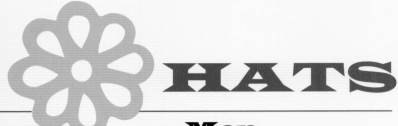

HATS

Men

The decade began well for men's hat manufacturers; men were rarely prepared to brave the outside world without a hat. Cloth caps were worn by the vast majority of working-class men for all occasions, and by middle- and upper-class men for sporting occasions, trilby-style hats being worn by them for the rest of the time. The exceptions

younger man. Details are a cut-edge felt which shows to the full the upsweep of the brim. The model has a narrow band and a tapering crown. Colour trends will include new shades of green, grey, and brown. The 1960 Tyrolean style is a new version of an old favourite which should also appeal to the younger man, whilst another new trend will be hats made from fabrics to match

Below left *In 1961, the large majority of men still wore hats outside.*
Below right *The comet had a narrow brim and a somewhat elaborate 'crest' at the side. April 1962.*

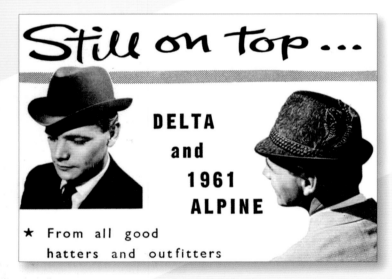

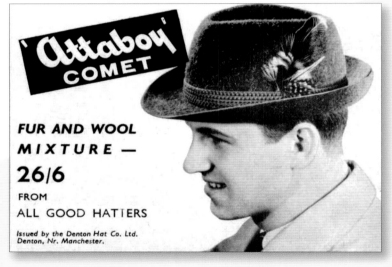

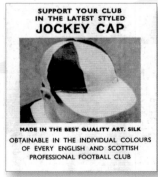

Above *The Jockey cap of 1965, an early version of the baseball cap.*

were the bowler, still the sign of the business man at work (or the artisan foreman among the working classes), and the top hat, worn only by diplomats, or at formal weddings, funerals and Ascot.

Yet change was in the air. **Men Only** in March 1960 predicted that there would be a trend to lightweight hats reflecting the fashion in suits. *'One, for casual wear, called the Week-Ender, weighs only 2oz. Another manufacturer has models claimed to be lighter than straw. Style trends in hats will include the Double Delta, the latest Delta shape. [The delta was a trilby-style hat popular in the 1950s.] This will suit the*

those of our town suits. Tweed hats are, of course, already being matched to sports jacket tweeds.'

Among young men, however, hat-wearing had become the exception. The heavily greased and shaped hair styles of the late 1950s would have been ruined by a hat, so most teenage boys went bareheaded.

The lightweight trend in hats continued, with **Men Only** reporting in July 1961: *'The trend in headwear this summer is to bright and lively hats, light in weight and cool to wear, made of straw, linen, felt or fabric. An eye-catcher for beach and holiday wear is a new Italian straw hat with a three-colour*

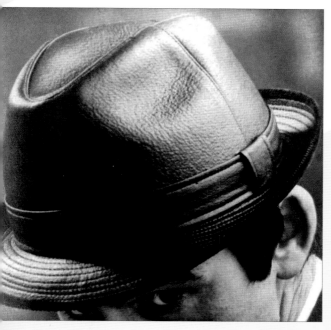

figures for last year show that the hat trend will continue. But there's still a long way to go. Townspeople generally seem less interested in hats than those who live in the country.'

The magazine continued: 'The biggest hope for the hat trade is the younger, bigger-headed generation, who have responded to the manufacturers' slow realization that something more than traditional British formality was needed to stimulate sales. That interesting ingredient called style. There was the Mambo, then the Robin Hood. In its turn came the Delta, probably the industry's staple line today. The most recent fashion hit is the Comet, with its rakish Edwardian look. Manufacturers are

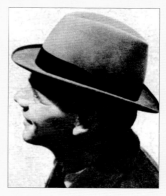

Far left November 1969. A version of the mods' pork pie' hat, made in 'Buflex'.

Above October 1961. Homburg-style hat, but with the fashionable narrow brim of the period.

plaited band and two miniature wine bottles as ornament. It should be in the shops this month selling at around a guinea.'

In October the magazine reported that 'the Comet is the name given to the new style of semi-formal hat for this winter. A feature is the changed crown shape – both back and front taper steeply back towards each other. It has a narrow brim with sleek side curl, to give an overall silhouette more streamlined than the Delta.

'Reminiscent of the Regency style of headwear, the Comet will be available in several variations including the newest version of the Homburg in a light grey fur felt, with a flat brim curled over with a lip. The Comet, like its predecessors the Robin Hood, the Delta and the Alpine, is not the brand name of any one manufacturer.'

In 1962 all still seemed well; indeed, as **Men Only** reported in April, hatters were hoping to increase business. 'British men are still not as hat-conscious as the hatters would like them to be – although about 68 per cent are estimated to be regular hat-wearers. Business is improving, however. In 1960 hatters did record trade – more than 2,500,000 hats sold – and provisional

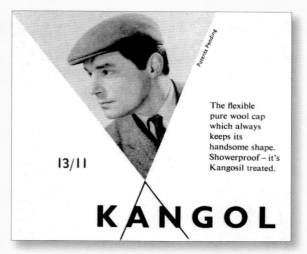

13/11

The flexible pure wool cap which always keeps its handsome shape. Showerproof – it's Kangosil treated.

Patents Pending

KANGOL

finding definite colour preferences. Browns and the lighter shades of green seem to be popular, while blue and grey seem to have gone out of favour – for the time being at least. The most likely new trend is American-influenced Gun Club. It features a narrow snap brim, wider bands and a tapering crown, which is likely to become rather higher later in the year.'

Despite the hope that the younger generation would take up the hat-wearing habit, they stubbornly refused to do so, and even more disastrously for the hat trade the 1960s revolution in fashion was starting. The fashionable look was a determinedly youthful one – and wearing hats had come

Left The cloth cap, worn by the working class everyday, and by the middle and upper classes as casual wear. April 1962.

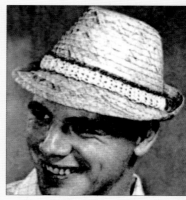

Above Raffia beach hat 'in the latest Alpine shape', May 1961.

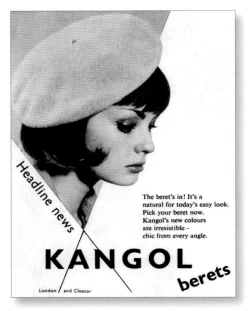

The beret's in! It's a natural for today's easy look. Pick your beret now. Kangol's new colours are irresistible – chic from every angle.

Headline news

KANGOL berets

London and Cleator

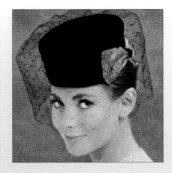

to be seen as something that only old men did. The new US president John F. Kennedy fuelled this reaction against hat-wearing; he hated wearing one, and was hardly ever photographed in one. If you ever see a photograph of him in a hat, he is almost unrecognisable.

With the onset of the swinging mid-1960s, when anything went and the more way out the better, hats made occasional comebacks, especially the more old-fashioned styles, such as top hats or bowlers, which might indeed be worn with military-style uniforms. Another such fashion was for the Russian-style fur hat. In April 1968 **Men Only** asked, *'Could it be that the tendency for men to wear fur hats over the last few years arises out of more than a simple fashion fad? Might we be treading steadily back to a fashion period which will require heavier materials again, and even a possible resuscitation of the hat industry?'*

Women

As with men, hat-wearing became a sign of the diverging generations at the start of the 1960s. Most younger women rarely wore hats; this had a lot to do with the fashionable hairstyles of the period, many of which were piled high into a beehive or bird's nest, making hat wearing difficult. One way to deal with this was to wear a hat in the form of a high, rather shapeless flowerpot, but it was not a good look.

One of the most fashionable hat designers at that time was the Dane Aage Thaarup, who made some of the queen's hats. When asked how the spring models of 1960 should be worn, he replied that *'they call for poise and a certain amount of grooming, but will suit the Englishwoman perfectly. Very ladylike, calling for effort,*

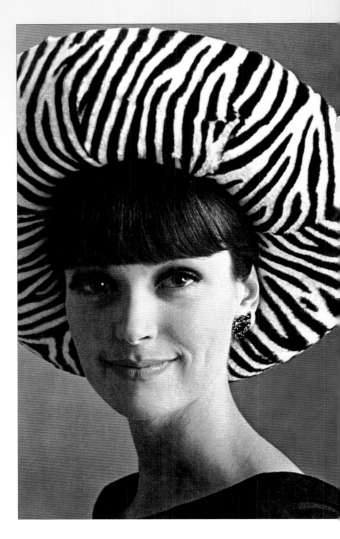

because the hair at the back shows. No more hiding your hair under a bucket!'

Of course, your size and shape dictated the type of hat you should wear, and magazines gave advice on the subject. **Housewife** in October 1961: *'The taller woman's choice of hats is practically limitless, with only one real exception – the sky-high crown.... The full-figured woman can balance her silhouette with stand-away necklines and unfussy, large hats – a full length mirror will immediately tell her whether or not the proportion of her to the rest of her outfit is correct.'* And for the short woman: *'Hats should be small head-huggers, and continue upwards to add to the general illusion of height.'* That year's **Boyfriend Annual** expanded: *'Large ones do not suit the small girl – they make her look*

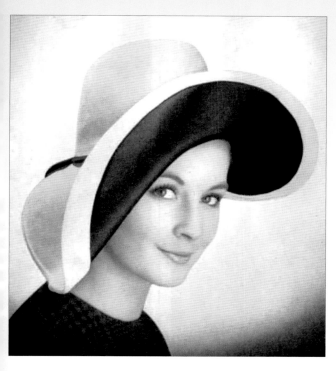

like a mushroom. So if you buy a hat see that it balances your shape. High crowns will give you height, but don't let the hat be too broad.'

For many young women, it became smart to wear a headscarf; hats were only worn for special occasions, and were often designed to accommodate the high hairstyles, with deep roomy crowns. In 1962, there was a brief revival of 1930s fashions, signalled by a return of the beret and the cloche.

Top left *The elaborately large hat of the 1950s still flourished in June 1961.*

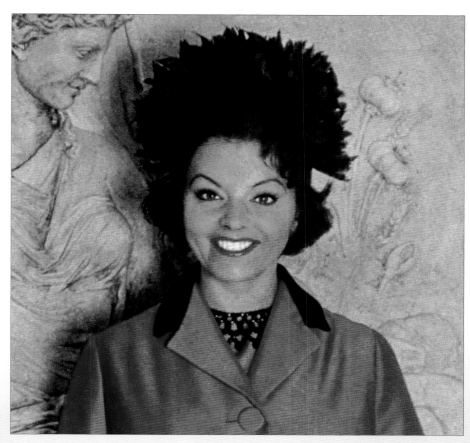

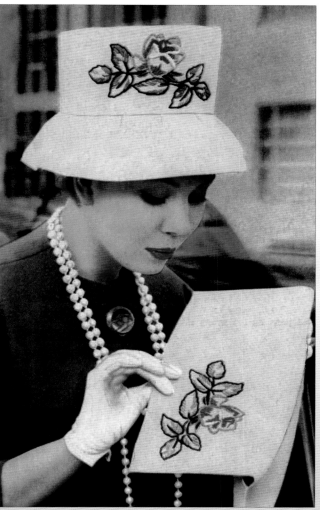

Other popular styles in the early 1960s were wide-brimmed sombreros, chrysanthemum-shaped concoctions made up of lots of petals, and the pillbox. These could be attached to the back of a built-up hairstyle, and were made popular by JFK's wife, so much so that they were often referred to as Jackie Kennedy hats.

Courrèges' highly influential Space Age collection of 1964 included high-domed, helmet-style hats, and the style, dubbed the 'bathing cap', was much copied and adapted

Above *Large flower-style hats were popular in spring/summer 1963.*

Lower left *A 'flower-pot' hat, 'with matching bag, July 1963.*

Far right *Striking fur hood, January 1969.*

over the next few years, with close-fitting, Victorian-style boys' caps, flying helmets and jockey caps all popular, as well as small berets and helmets perched well forward on the brow.

A variation of the space helmet was the hood. **Woman's Own** in October 1966 gave directions for making one in fun-fur leopard skin *(shown below)*.

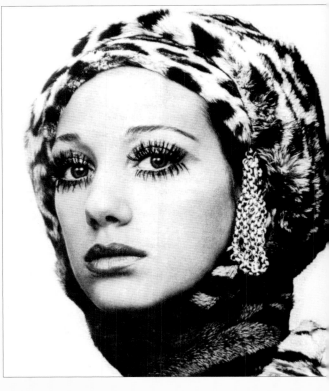

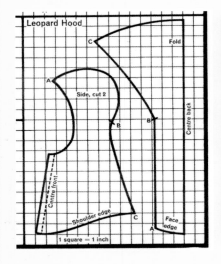
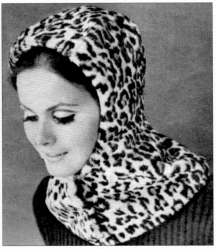

'*Materials: ¾yd. fur fabric, ¾yd. lining, 3 poppers.*
Join sides to back A-B-C. Join lining the same way. With right sides of fabric and lining together, machine round face edge, shoulder edge, and one side of front edge. Clip, turn out and press all edges. Slip-stitch open front edge together. Sew poppers at centre front edge of hood.'

nautical styles complete with pom-poms.

As with men's hats, women's hats went through a rather bizarre stage, with deerstalkers, top hats and bowlers all having their day. **Woman** magazine in September 1967 told its readers that the latest hats '… *highlight the wide-brimmed look, bowlers and highway-woman hats; peaked caps and man-type trilbies, often with buckles or ribbon trims.*' One such fashion which stuck was the Cossack-style fur hat, popular with both men and women. The influential film **Bonnie and Clyde** also premiered in 1967 and this resulted in a new lease of life for the beret and the cloche.

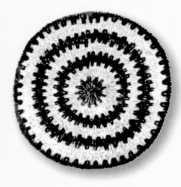

Above *A crocheted beret from January 1966.*

Right *Hippy-style hat, August 1969.*

Another variation was the Breton sailor's cap, made popular by the folk singer, Donovan. The cap was one of his trademarks, and it rapidly became known as the Donovan cap. **Rave** magazine in May 1965 told its readers that '*John Michael are making them in denim. John Stephen in linen.*'

In turn, the beret blended with the cap giving rise to far larger caps, butcher-boy caps, Tam o'Shanters and

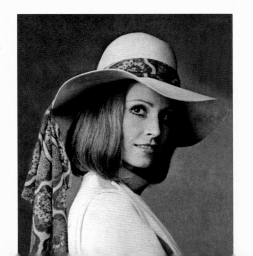

These styles then gave way to a new look that would dominate the last two years of the decade. Epitomised by Biba, it was romantic, mysterious and flowing, and it inspired the resurgence of hat-wearing as a popular fashion in the form of furs, berets and large, floppy hats.

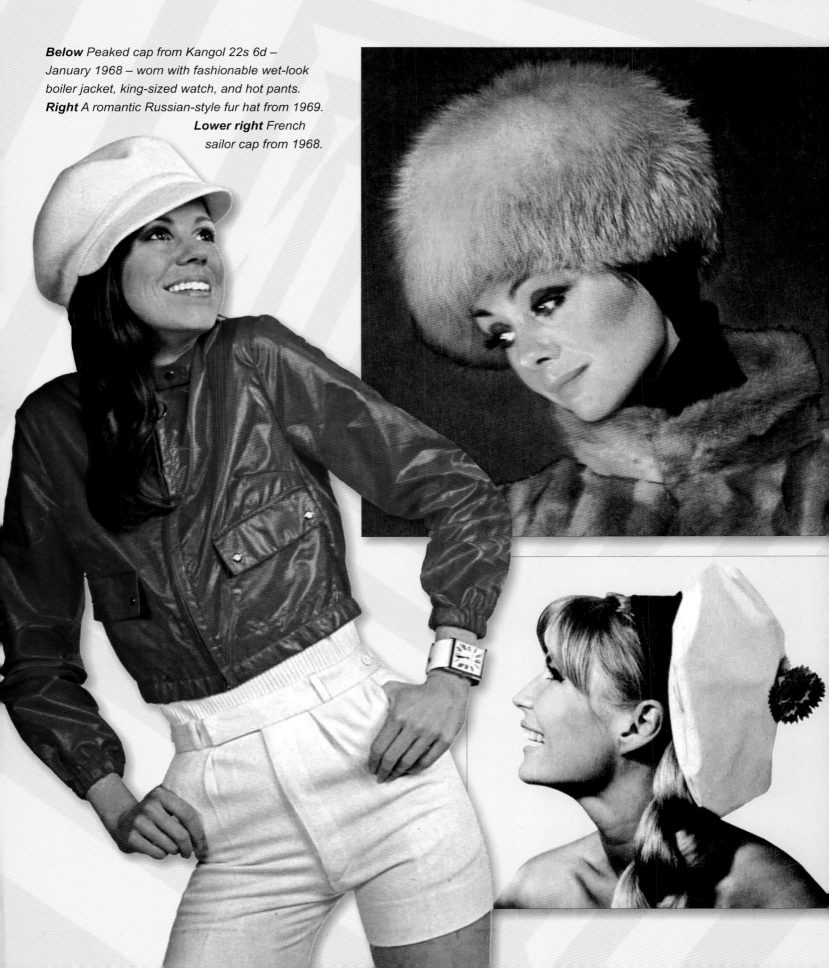

Below *Peaked cap from Kangol 22s 6d – January 1968 – worn with fashionable wet-look boiler jacket, king-sized watch, and hot pants.*
Right *A romantic Russian-style fur hat from 1969.*
Lower right *French sailor cap from 1968.*

GLOVES

Right June 1960, At the start of the decade, women still routinely wore gloves for any formal, or even semi-formal occasion.

Below June 1961, long gloves were still the height of elegance for evening wear.

For cold weather most gloves were made of knitted wool, either hand knitted or more likely machine-knitted, although other materials, such as leather, sheepskin and man-made fibres, were fairly common.

Fashion, however, dictated if and when gloves should be worn at other times. At the beginning of the 1960s, it was still very much the thing for a woman to wear gloves on any occasion that required dressing up, such as going out on social or formal occasions. It was also still regarded as smart for men to wear gloves on such occasions, but not to the same extent.

For women formal occasions, or evening wear, demanded the wearing of long, elbow-length gloves in suede or leather in cold temperatures, or silk, satin, nylon or similar during the summer months. Shorter 'bracelet-length' gloves were also acceptable, often edged with fur. **Modern Woman** in December 1964 informed its readers: *'The latest trend from Paris is for gloves matching your ensemble – even in jewel-bright shades. This applies particularly if*

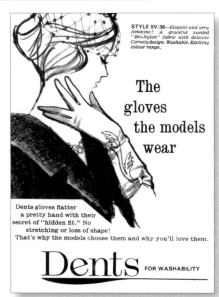

STYLE 5V/38—*Elegant and very feminine! A graceful sueded "Bri-Nylon" fabric with delicate Cornely design. Washable. Exciting colour range.*

The gloves the models wear

Dents gloves flatter a pretty hand with their secret of "hidden fit." No stretching or loss of shape! That's why the models choose them and why you'll love them.

Dents FOR WASHABILITY

the sleeve is fashionably trimmed with fur. Don't just tone in the glove or you will have a three-shaded arm. And remember, gloves can complete an outfit or absolutely ruin it. Points to bear in mind: a lady does not take off her gloves to shake hands (unless they are muddy gardening gloves) but always removes them for eating.'

As the style swung violently towards the young and informal, glove wearing went totally out of fashion, except in one area – driving gloves. As the number of cars, and therefore drivers, soared, the fashion for car coats and driving gloves likewise grew. And not everyone wearing a car coat or driving gloves even owned a car!

Driving gloves, indeed all gloves, benefited from the advances being made in the use of leather. As it became thinner and more colourful, so leather gloves began to appear in a wide range of primary colours in line with the fashions of the time.

Driving gloves, inspired by a fashion for cutaway sections in women's fashions generally, evolved from a standard glove shape, with leather palms and knitted backs, to the cutaway glove which soon established itself as the standard.

Gloves became a fun accessory, with short stretch gloves available in checks or stripes, and long leather or wet-look plastic

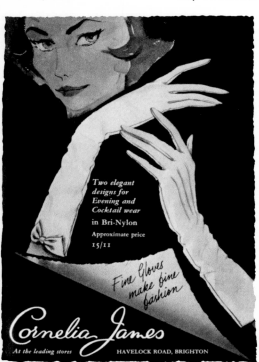

Two elegant designs for Evening and Cocktail wear in Bri-Nylon
Approximate price 15/11

Fine Gloves make fine fashion

Cornelia James
At the leading stores HAVELOCK ROAD, BRIGHTON

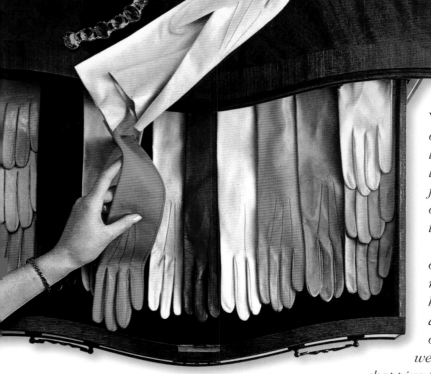

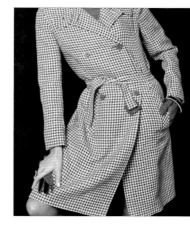

Left April 1965. A good example of the wide range of bright colours available in leather gloves.

Above The driving glove as pure fashion, combining bright colours, and the 'cut-away'. January 1966.

gloves to match long 'kinky boots'.

With the arrival of Op Art fashions, **Woman** in October 1965 recommended '*harlequin stretch-nylon gloves*' at 12s 11d a pair, while **Vanity Fair** in January 1966 advised its readers to '*wear black and white gloves, decorated but not gaudy. The three above are all by Kir. From left to right. White kid with a slim vent edged with black, 42s. Black fabric with two white leather stripes, 10s 6d. Black fabric with white leather to trim the cuff, 12s 11d.*'

Woman magazine in September 1967 told its readers about the latest fashions: '*Cut-out gloves continue for sporty wear with popper fastenings, driving versions, often demi-fingered. The stud story with nailhead trims too, appears on gloves. Most practical: the glove with ring-zip up the centre front.*'

With the coming of the romantic look in the late 1960s, both men and women could once again wear more formal gloves, but for some the social nuances of glove-wearing

had been lost. A reader asked **Woman's Journal** in 1969: '*Two or three social functions are looming ahead and I would like to know what gloves to buy for day and evening and what one is expected to do with them?*'

The reply was: '*Wear them out of doors if for no other reason than to keep your hands warm. But as a fashion accessory they are currently out of style, meaning that once we wore them even when shopping for groceries; now it's on with the false eyelashes instead, before facing the world. On the other hand there are occasions when we must comply with convention: a wedding, reception or a big dinner. Always buy the best (French) and stick to white, champagne and all shades of beige. When you arrive at your destination, take them off and hold them with your bag, park them if you leave your coat, or, at an evening dinner, you can leave them with your bag on a sofa or chair. But don't put them in your bag. And never eat in the things.*'

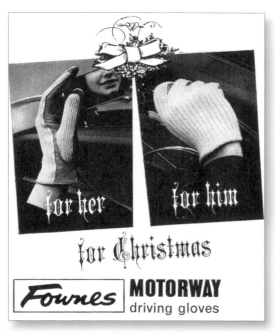

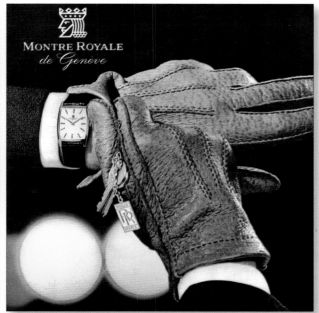

Above Driving gloves from 1964 and 1969, for 'him', for 'her', and the upwardly mobile!

BELTS

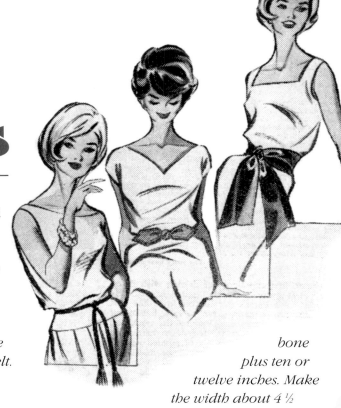

Right A selection of DIY belts from June 1961, directions on how to make are within the text.

Below 'Easy "in" to the New look, key on thigh-length chain, and; fringed suede belt to tie, luxuriously, on simple dress. Child's play to make. Choose cream to contrast with grey or aubergine with pink.' October 1965.

In June 1961 **Woman's Weekly** gave its readers instructions for making belts, and at the same time it revealed some interesting insights into fashionable belts and how they were worn. *'Good belts are expensive. Yet one with character can make your dress, especially the simple, straight ones which are fashionable this summer. If you alter an old dress into the new gym-tunic style, you'll still need a belt. So make one yourself – and here's how. Best-looking, most expensive, are those made of leather or suede, so if you have an oddment of either, treasure it. If positively no leather or suede is at hand, then use satin-finished elasticised fabric or even felt in any of the brilliant colours and back it so that it won't stretch.'*

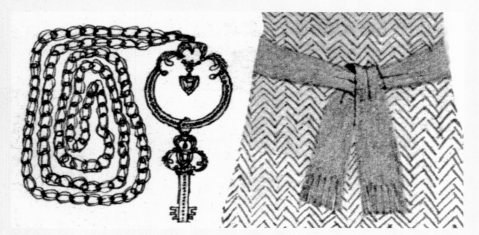

'As you know, the smart way to wear a belt today is just on the hip-bone, loose and casual-looking and not tightly buckled at the waist. So the belt will have to be longer, especially as the newest style is to wear it tied in a knot or lapped over. You'll need it about 36 inches long – or more accurately, the measurement round the top of your hip-bone plus ten or twelve inches. Make the width about 4 ½ inches (⅛ yard if you're buying) which allows for a turning on to the lining.

'If the dress material is not too thick, use it for the lining and choose a strong, brilliant colour for the belt itself. Make a knot in front and catch the stay, allowing the two ends to drop to unequal lengths. In order not to disturb the knot at each wearing, make a hook and eye fastening at one side. Do not use stiffening, only the lining.

'The double knot – As a change from long hanging ends, tie the lined strip in a double knot in front, with longish ends taken back at each side and stitched invisibly to the belt. Here you can make an opening behind the knot, so there is no need to have a side fastening. Mitre each end, stitching all round at the same time as you do the sides.

'Last, you simply must have a bootlace belt. Cut a long length 1 ½ inches wide, lay cotton wool along the middle in a strip and roll the sides of the fabric together, catching with small stitches in matching cotton. Cut a strip of fringed self fabric and roll round each end of the bootlace. Knot to tie.

'Many dresses this season have a seam across the hipline. No reason why you can't wear a belt – but better not a wide, conspicuous one if you are definitely on the short side. The single knot with long unequal ends or the double knot with ends stitched back on to the belt itself. Which will suit you? It depends if you're the casual type, or a neat, orderly kind of person.'

The **Boyfriend Annual** also gave advice on how a belt could make the most of your shape: *'If you're thin this probably means you have a waist that other girls are madly envious about. So wear wide belts that show up that wasp waist.'* In 1962 the waist returned as part of a fashionable dress shape, and it was emphasised by large, tight belts.

With the arrival of the little girl look came wide belts in bold colours, which added to the impression of extreme shortness that typified the 'pelmet' miniskirt. In 1965 chains became the height of fashion, and a chain belt was a must.

In September 1967 **Woman** magazine reported on the latest fashions. *'Belt – back with a bang, waist-whittling, studded with nails, perforated and horse brass buckle fastened. Buckles dull and oxidized. Most fun belt – a suede one reversing to a tape measure. New, too, is the printed newspaper belt. Also the watch chain belt with coloured face watch.'*

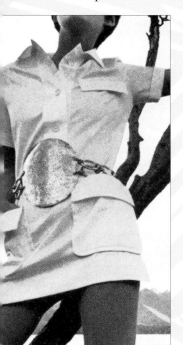

Above *As minis got smaller, so belts tended to get bigger, this from May 1968.*
Right *A selection of fashionable belts from 1968.*

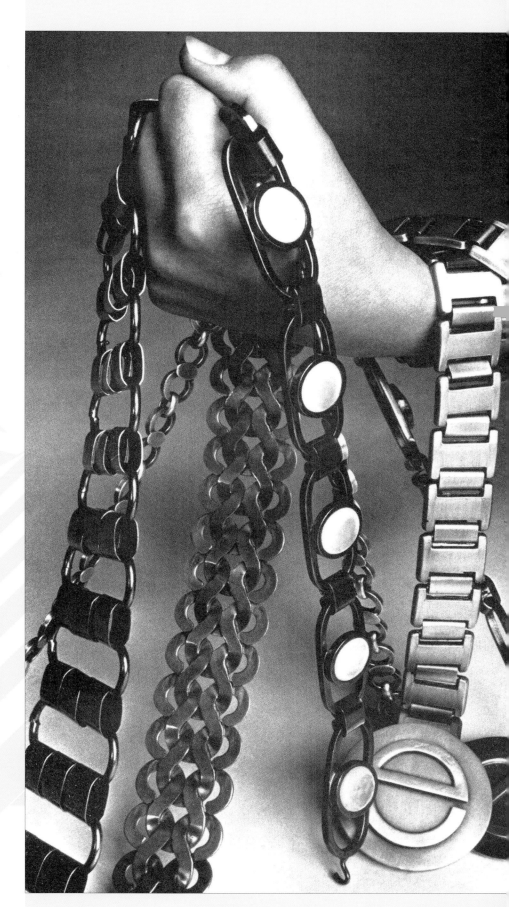

BAGS, LUGGAGE AND UMBRELLAS

Bags

At the start of the 1960s the most popular handbag was large, rectangular, and most fashionably made of mock or (if you could afford it) real crocodile, snake or lizard skin. They were, however, a practical item, capacious enough to carry lots of things and, if required in emergency, an effective weapon!

As the decade wore on, bags became smaller and brighter, in tune with the fashions of the time.

Up till now baskets had generally been used for shopping, but they were somewhat unwieldy and lacked the fashionable look. Their place was taken by raffia bags, or the more modern string bag. **Woman's Realm** in March 1963 gave the following advice: *'When using a string bag for shopping, I line it with an ordinary polythene bag. It keeps the contents dry on a rainy day and prevents small items from slipping through the mesh.'*

Handbags remained fairly large, but softer, brightly coloured leather was used to great effect, while the old rigid rectangular profile was changing.

Smaller bags in leather, or the new plastic imitation leather, became popular, as did suede, fake fur and even upholstery material. Smaller bags could be made as shoulder bags, and many had both a handle and a shoulder strap.

By the middle of the decade fashions were changing rapidly, and the wilder the look the better. In January 1966 **Vanity Fair** advised its readers to *'have a quilted handbag with beads stitched into the quilting, and chain handles.'*

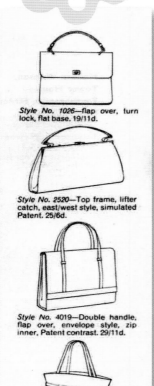

Style No. 1026—flap over, turn lock, flat base. 19/11d.

Style No. 2520—Top frame, lifter catch, east/west style, simulated Patent. 25/6d.

Style No. 4019—Double handle, flap over, envelope style, zip inner, Patent contrast. 29/11d.

Style No. 4020—Soft pouchy, two handles, Dorothy style, top entry zip. 29/11d.

Style No. 8008—adjustable shoulder strap, inner zip pocket, flat base. 39/11d.

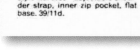

Above *A selection of bags from December 1963.*

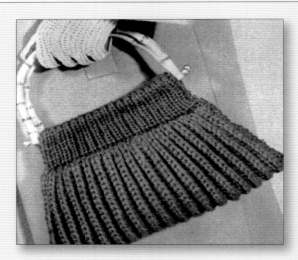

Modern Woman magazine in November 1964 revealed how to make a knitted handbag *(shown above)* in an evening:
'Materials: 4ozs. Lee Target Fleetknit, a pair each of Nos.1 and 5 knitting needles, a piece of Vilene, approximately 14in x 16in lining. A pair of handles with removable metal bars.
Tension: 3 sts. to 1 inch
Cast on 40 sts. on No.5 needles and work in k. 1, p. 1 rib for 20 rows. Change to No. 1 needles and ptn. 1st row: – *K. into st. below st. on left needle. p. 1; rep. from * to end. Rep. this row for 11 1/2 ins. Change to No.5 needles and work 20 rows in k. 1. p. 1 rib. Cast off.
TO MAKE UP: Press lightly. Cut Vilene to shape and size of bag, cut lining, allowing 1/2in turnings all round. Sew in Vilene, leaving 1 7/8in unlined (ribbed borders); sew in lining, turning in edges all round. Fold ribbed borders over bars of handles; stitch. Sew up side seams, leaving borders open.'

Along with the fashion for crocheted dresses came crocheted berets and swimming costumes, and in September 1967, **Stitchcraft** gave instructions for making a 'Crochet Bag' (shown below).

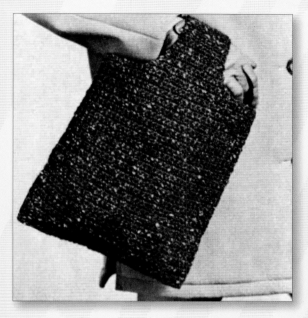

'Materials: 5 (1oz.) balls Patons Bracken Double Knitting.
No.6 crochet hook.
Piece of buckram, 10 x 32in.
3/8yd. 36in wide lining material.
Measurements: Length from top of handle, 16in.; width, 10½in.
Tension: 3 1/2 d.c. to an inch.
Abbreviations: ch. = chain; d.c. = double crochet.
Make 38 ch. 1st row: miss 1 ch. from hook (this counts as 1st d.c.). 36 d.c. in 36 ch., turn with 1 ch.
2nd row: miss 1st d.c., 36 d.c., turn with 1 ch.
Rep. 2nd row until work measures 11½in, then shape for handles.
Next 2 rows: work to last 9 d.c., turn. Now work 1 d.c. less at each end of next 5 rows.
Continue straight on remaining sts. for a further 3in. Fasten off.
Make another piece the same. Press parts on wrong side under a damp cloth.

Join halves together along lower edge and press seam.
Cut buckram to fit shape, 1/8in less all round than crochet fabric opened out flat.
Cut lining 1in larger than buckram, then turn spare material over stiffening and tack; machine in position close to edge.
Pin stiffening to crochet and slip-stitch, then fold bag and join sides and top of handle. Slip-stitch edges of linings together at back of handle.'

Below The Mrs. Thatcher-style bag, November 1962.

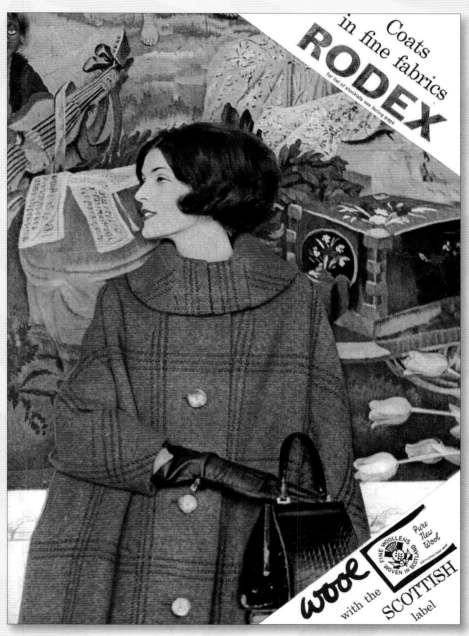

Coats in fine fabrics **RODEX**
for list of stockists see facing page

FINE WOOLLENS WOVEN IN SCOTLAND
Pure New Wool

Wool with the **SCOTTISH** label

Far right With the advent of the youth look, bags got much smaller and brighter, October 1963.

Below 'Plastic formula fabrics', in other words imitation leather, were as popular as the real thing. April 1966.

At the same time **Woman** magazine described the latest fashions, and it had this to say on the subject: *'Bags – bolder, more capacious, more practical, with horsey trims. Enter the briefcase-cum-bag, the mini-trunk.'*

With the hippy fashion came huge canvas bags, or tapestry bags, often fringed or embroidered, and ex-army shoulder bags.

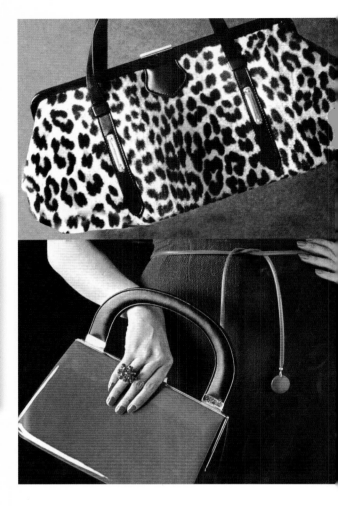

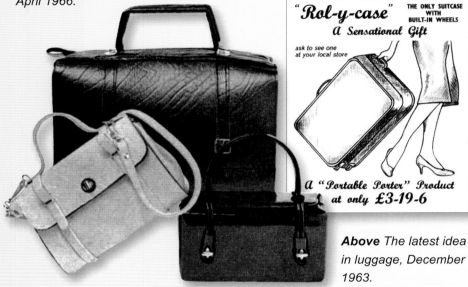

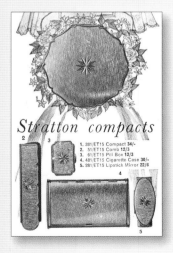

Above Handbag accessories, Autumn 1965.

Above The latest idea in luggage, December 1963.

The heavy make-up worn by the mid-1960s dolly bird meant that her handbag always contained a good supply of cosmetics, certainly a compact and a lipstick at the very least.

Previously no man would have been seen dead with a bag. Various men's designers had tried to introduce handbags, but they met with little success even when they were rebranded as the man bag. However, many more people were now taking part in sports and this meant that a sports-type holdall became quite acceptable.

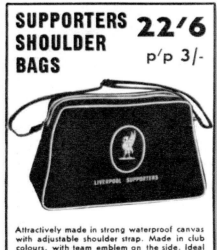

Suitcases

The huge increase in people taking holidays, especially foreign holidays, meant that the old cardboard and fibre suitcases fell out of fashion.

New materials, especially plastics and fibreglass were used to create modern-looking, light, bright luggage.

As with clothes, imitation leather was popular, even fashionable, although the real thing was preferred by those with the cash to afford it.

Left Men could get away with carrying this sort of holdall in 1969.

Umbrellas

The ever-quickening pace of change in the fashion world tended to prove very expensive for the consumer, but a good dress could be made to last by the addition of accessories in the latest styles or colours. The umbrella – often a necessity in rainy Britain – was perfect in this respect.

Umbrellas came in all the latest styles and colours: in wet-look plastic, in Op Art and psychedelic patterns and colours, even in silver when that briefly became fashionable. At first the telescopic umbrella was all the rage, with its ultra-modern Space-Age feel, but as the fashion for the Edwardian look took hold, men favoured a retrun to the old-fashioned rolled brolly, as sported by Steed in the popular TV programme, **The Avengers**.

Below Samsonite solid cases from May 1968.

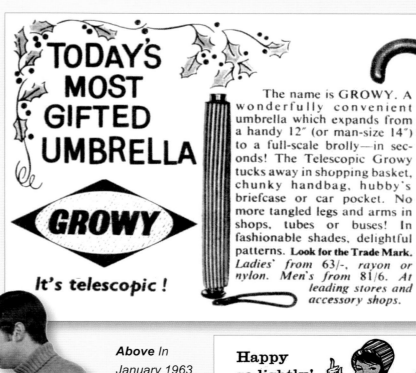

Above In January 1963 the latest thing was the telescopic umbrella.

Right Luggage in June 1961.

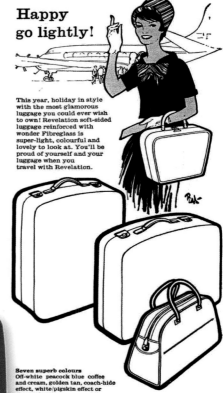

SPECTACLES

Right Cats-eyes were not dead. These are an interesting combination of fifties' shape and sixties' solid frames. September 1967.

Below Women's frames from May 1965. The 'Caine' referred to in the top is, of course, Michael Caine, one of the heart-throb actors of the time.

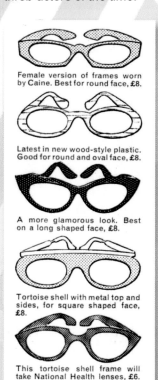

Female version of frames worn by Caine. Best for round face, £8.

Latest in new wood-style plastic. Good for round and oval face, £8.

A more glamorous look. Best on a long shaped face, £8.

Tortoise shell with metal top and sides, for square shaped face, £8.

This tortoise shell frame will take National Health lenses, £6.

Fashionable spectacles at the start of the decade had a more restrained, softer look than had been the case in the 1950s. Thus, the extremely angular, jewelled cat's-eye glasses for women were replaced by a combination frame – a wire lower half with a plastic upper bar and sides. For men, the more fashionable frames were still made in solid black plastic, but the hard square shape of the 1950s became rounder and softer.

Everywoman in April 1961 reviewed the fashion in spectacles: *'With so many types of specs to suit every shape of face there's no excuse for not choosing a good-looks asset. In deciding, first consider your contour. Only long or squarish faces can take deep lenses. Eyebrows matter. Whether you show them or not, the upper rim of the frame should follow the natural arch. Colour matters. If you can afford only one pair, choose it in basic sherry, "smoke", or black – plain or two-toned. Generally, brunettes can carry off the most exciting colours. And on close-set eyes keep colour concentrated on the outer corners. Occasion matters. Décolleté necklines need delicate eye-frames. If you're a party-goer, choose a slim outline for day-into-evening wear.'*

Woman magazine in October 1963 took a similar line: *'There's a positive galaxy of gorgeous frame shapes and shades available, and a perfect pair for any girl who's prepared to put in a little time*

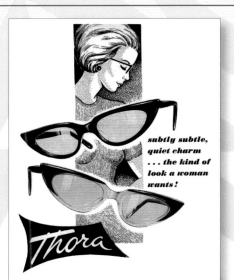

subtly subtle, quiet charm . . . the kind of look a woman wants!

Thora

picking and choosing.

'Glasses can do a great deal to improve looks. Gently-rounded frames can actually soften sharp features. A "snub" nose can be given the illusion of length via glasses with a high, slender bridge: and a long nose shortened with a bridge that's low-placed. An elongated upper frame helps slim a broad forehead, and heavier emphasis here than on the lower part of the frame will balance up a wide jawline and narrow forehead. Full faces look slim with wide frames without depth, while chunky frames, deep lenses, give long faces the instant shortening treatment!

'But glasses can do more than this. They can bring out your true personality. Delicate frame tones – lilacs, corals, pale blues and greens – emphasize a blonde's femininity. Big, bold frames suggest that there's more to a shy-looking girl than actually meets the eye! Darker and more vivid colours lend brunettes vibrancy, and light up a warm-toned skin. Tortoiseshell tones can look tops on redheads! The latest trend is to team frame colours with the clothes you wear – the girl who looks stunning in a scarlet dress will find matching frames a flattering accessory.'

Bifocals and even trifocals were available, and in 1964 Norville's introduced a varifocal lens, *'Varilux the lens of the future – Now'*.

The emphasis on eyes in make-up created a fashion for large round frames, known as owl eyes. Half-moon frames for reading were also popular in a range of colours and styles, including a semi-cat's-eye, marquesite model.

Rave magazine in May 1965 declared that: *'What spectacles can do for a man, they can do for a girl too. They can make you look more striking, give you added appeal and a touch of glamour. See Michael Caine. Yes, for summer sixty-five, glasses are goffy. [With it.]*

'Once upon a time glasses made a girl feel unattractive – the frames were all very plain and practical looking – even the most fabulous girls could feel awkward in plastic pink! But today it's a different story. During the last few years spectacle frames have been revolutionised to the extent that now girls and, indeed, boys often wear specs for

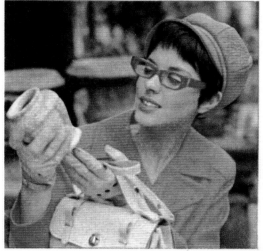

◄ MASTERLY MATCH

Bold red frames match suit and hat. Shallow lenses are framed in transparent plastic, laminated with colour. Sides are hinged high on temple to preserve a shallow line.

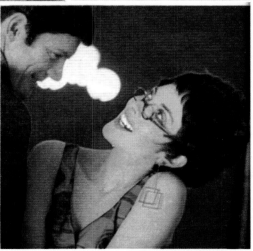

DISCOTHEQUE ► DATE

Mini "granny" specs with tortoiseshell plastic frames. Strictly for fun, they're a copy of the Victorian reading glasses that grandma used to wear.

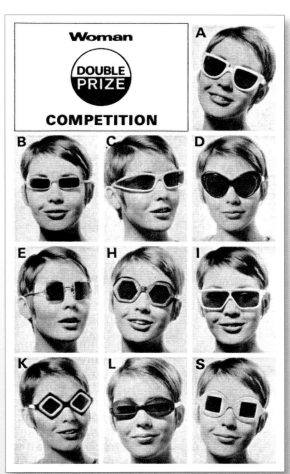

Above Some very 'groovy' sunglasses by Correna, June 1967.

effect only. Many people do look more striking in a dramatic pair of spectacles! A couple of years ago it was the "Buddy Holly" look specwise; last year the big round "Lolita" look; early this year "in" girls have been wearing the old-fashioned "granny" frames. Now oval frames seem specially popular. It is very important to choose your frames according to the shape of your face and eyes and also to the spacing of your eyes and eyebrows. The top line of the frames should follow the curves of the brows – if they are higher or lower at any point they look odd and heavy. Really fashionable frames are rather expensive costing from about £6 up. But I'm afraid National Health frames understandably are not very fashion conscious. Nevertheless the plain

Above Women's fashion frames, including the 'granny' below, July 1967.

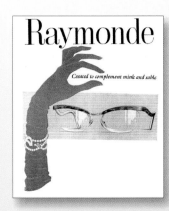

Above A 1961 softened 'composite' form of the fifties cats-eye glasses.

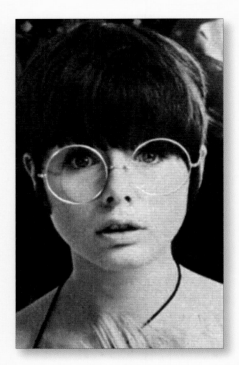

Above Owl-eye glasses from January 1969.

rounded frames are available in a selection of colours and cost about £1 17s complete with lenses.

'For girls who can't wear glasses because of the work they do, like modelling or acting, contact lenses are an excellent investment. Not everyone can wear lenses but the initial test with either your optician or the clinic to which he sends you will answer that one. If you are given the okay you'll need five to six fittings after which the lenses will fit you perfectly. They can be painful in the early stages but if you persevere most people can wear them easily without irritation. Contact lenses cost from 35 guineas including the treatment fee.'

For men, the fashionable shape was a square or rounded square frame. In 1964–5 this had usually been made of gold-coloured metal, but in late 1965 this was superseded by solid black or dark brown plastic, as worn by film star Michael Caine.

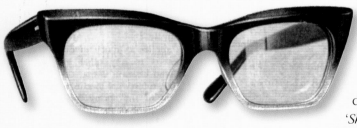

Above These frames came in 'Black Solid, Sherry two-tone, Smoke two-tone' - March 1969.

In July 1967 **Woman** magazine declared that: 'Shape's the big news in specs this year. Newest sun specs are frankly fun, but the biggest trend – in both plain and tinted specs – is towards a soft feminine look. The man-size squares, the big, bold owl eyes are slimmer, curvier – easier to wear for most. When it comes to shape, the choice is bigger than ever before.

'Colour matters, but choice of frame shape and colour could be even bigger – ophthalmic and dispensing opticians naturally stock frames to meet demand. If you're after something different, tell him – the chances are he can get it for you. But remember not all prescription lenses will fit all frames, and the practitioner's main consideration is your sight, so take his advice. As a general colour guide, deeper tones, dark reds, blues, browns and ebony flatter brunettes. Lighter shades complement fair hair but a dark-eyed blonde can look great in darker frames.'

The **Optician** in July 1969 commented that '…the ladies are wearing the trousers and the men are growing their hair to shoulder length (or almost). The traditional visual difference between the sexes is fast disappearing – to state the obvious, and the effect of the change upon spectacle makers can be seen by scanning their catalogues.

'Black square frames for men, black almost square frames for women – gold-filled combination frames for men, the same with minor differences for women. All-gold-filled frames for men (which have been popular for quite a while now) are now followed by all-gold-filled frames for women.'

Sunglasses

Hitherto sunglasses had primarily been a functional item, worn only occasionally in this country. This meant that they were normally cheap and cheerful in appearance. But as the habit of taking summer holidays grew in popularity, and particularly holidays abroad, sunglasses became part of a fashionable ensemble. **Woman's Realm** in May 1963 suggested that readers should: 'Give a bright look to earrings and frames of sunglasses by painting them to match with nail varnish. Pick a shade to go with your summer outfits.'

With the fashion focus moving to the eyes, glasses became an important accessory. **Rave** magazine in May 1965 informed its readers that 'Courrèges has some fantastic ideas. Like white sunglasses – even the lenses. Worn just for effect but what an effect. Glasses are right 'in' anyway. Boys have worn them, heavy-framed, to look terrific since last autumn. Now girls are doing it.'

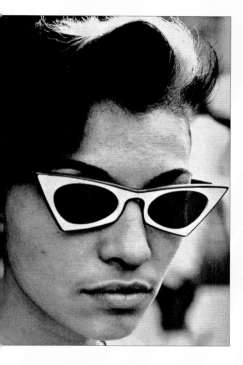

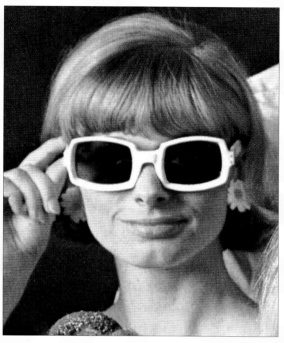

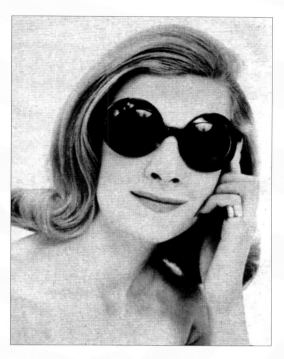

As fashions became more extreme, so did glasses. The most extreme 'fun' frames could be used for spectacles but cost deterred most women from purchasing expensive spectacles which would be out of fashion within a few weeks. However, for cheaper sunglasses, they were perfect. **Vanity Fair** in January 1966 advised readers to *'swap chic summer sunglasses for winter variations by Oliver Goldsmith, palely tinted in Winter Green, Winter Blue, Winter Brown, Winter Smoke and even Winter Pink, 6 guineas. To protect your eyes from very bright lights – or bright snow!*

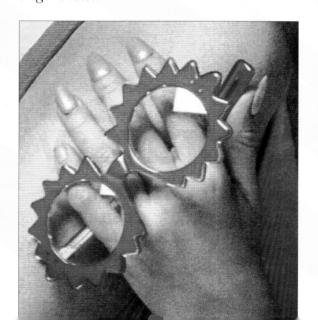

'Fun sunglasses with a wider lens to take over from the Courrèges fad. The top ones are in black and white and can be worn either way up as the bridge isn't set for any specific angle. 7 guineas. The lower pair are the chicest yet presentation of the steel-rimmed National Health look. They have subtle winter shades which make them perfect for indoors. 94s 6d. Both by Oliver Goldsmith.'

Woman magazine in May 1967 asked: *'Do you colour-match your sunglasses and earrings? It's a good idea, and soon they're selling ready-paired. "Sunsets" include specs, 2 guineas; earrings, 10s; ring, 7s 6d. Impact is Pow!'*

A reader wrote to **Woman** in August 1968: *'I was puzzled on holiday. I saw them on cords round necks. I saw them holding back hair; I saw them square, oval, triangular. Then I finally realized that they're no longer designed to keep sun out of eyes, sunglasses are accessories.'*

By 1969 Polaroid 'aviator' sunglasses, as worn by US pilots or Highway Patrolmen, were in style, especially those with mirrored lenses, as the fashion swung away from black plastic frames for men's spectacles towards wire frames.

Above, far left Very modernist sunglasses from 1961.
Above, centre In 1968 fashionable frames for both glasses and sunglasses were big, these from January.
Above right Continental style sunglasses from April 1961.

Far left 'Funky' frames for glasses or sunglasses, August 1968.

JEWELLERY

Men

At the start of the 1960s men wore little in the way of jewellery. Accepted accessories included cufflinks, and perhaps a tie pin and/or a signet ring, or wedding ring, rarely both.

With the exception of the tie pin, these conventions remained more or less unchanged until the advent of the hippies. As the widths of fashionable ties varied enormously from the narrow slim Jim to the exceptionally wide kipper, so the tie pin seemed out of place, either looking absurdly wide or ridiculously narrow. In its place came the tie tack, a pierced ear-type pin which was speared through the tie and fastened with a clip at the back. The clip

Below Cufflinks from December 1964.

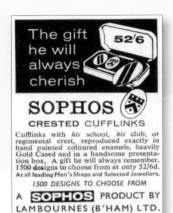

Above Select men and women's rings from the comfort of your own home in June 1961.
Far right A large selection of fashion jewellery, June 1961.

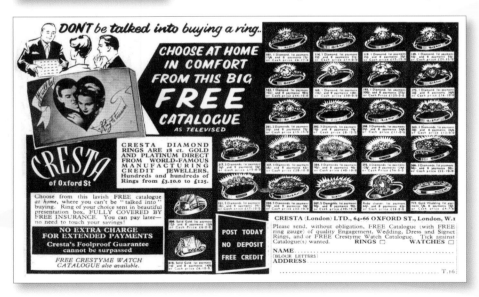

sometimes had a small chain attached, which could be passed through a shirt buttonhole, holding it in place.

With the advent of hippy fashions, men were free to wear far more jewellery, such as rows of beads, leather or beaded bracelets, peace bells and lots of rings.

Women

The most fashionable look in 1960 was a sophisticated one, and jewellery was worn in an unostentatious way. **Woman** magazine advised in February: *'Smooth as cream and simple as pie – that's the look of today's top model girls. Follow their example, cast aside baubles and beads and aim at that clear, uncluttered look to make you stand out in the crowd.*

'Dress extra carefully, put on your most professional make-up, then face the mirror without a single accessory. You look different, because now the accent is really on you – without frills.

'If you're sure that the picture is too

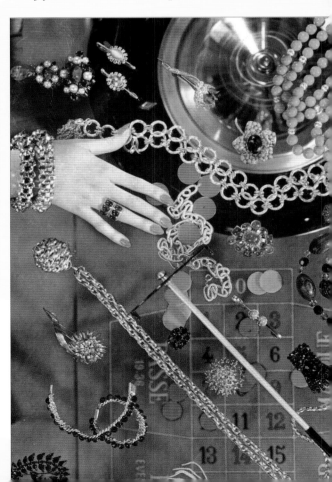

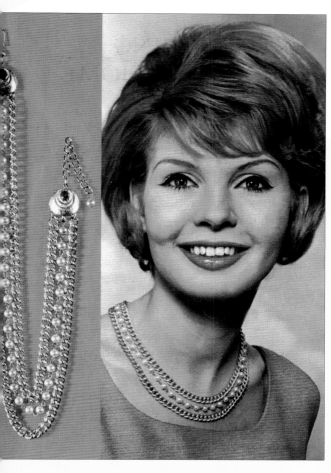

scale, with perhaps just one delicate piece to highlight a slim waist or an attractive shoulder line. The taller woman – dramatic jewellery is for her – row upon row of colourful beads; a giant brooch; huge rings.'

Chunky costume jewellery was very fashionable that year. The **Boyfriend Annual** advised its readers that 'If you're skinny ... You can look good in heavy chunky jewellery – particularly bangles and earrings. But avoid necklaces – they will draw attention to your thin neck.'

In 1963 the Swinging 1960s were dawning, but the basic rules had changed little, as this article from **Woman** magazine of November 1963 shows: 'Wear no more than two pieces of jewellery at a time. Say, brooch and bracelet or ring and necklace or brooch and ear-rings. Never ear-rings, brooch, necklace, bracelet and ring all at once. You might get away with it on Royal state occasions – but only if your jewels are real!

'Keep diamanté, showy, sparkly jewels and long ear-rings for after-six wear. Gilt,

stark, add tiny ear-rings or a slender bracelet. A touch more? Instead of adding another accessory, replace ear-rings with something larger, a chunkier bracelet. Ear-rings or bracelet or necklace or brooch. Well, maybe two sometimes. More very occasionally. All – never!'

Pearl necklaces had been very popular throughout the 1950s, and so they remained. **Woman's Weekly** in November 1960 advised that a necklace should complement your shape: 'If your neck is on the short side you shouldn't wind your beads too tightly. If you have too thin a neck, hollows at the base of the throat can be a problem, so cover them with a fashionable bib of beads when your dress has a cut-down neckline.'

Housewife in October 1961 reinforced the theme, recommending that for short women, 'Jewellery should be kept to a minimum and remain on the same small

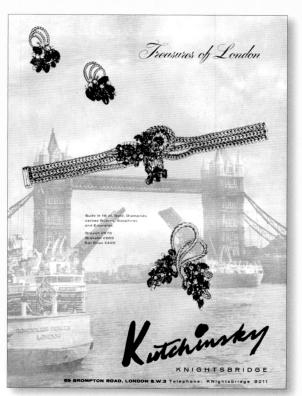

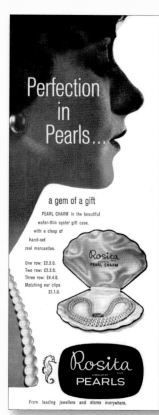

Left Costume necklace from April 1962.

Above Pearls were a traditionally perennial gift, these from June 1961.

Left In the early sixties, jewellery was either precious metal and stones, or imitation, costume jewellery. This from June 1961.

Right *Black and white plastic jewellery was perfect for the op art fashion, 1968.*

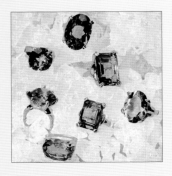

Above *Citrine Quartz solitaires by Karatclad, October 1966.*

Below *Dangly earrings in plastic, it's October 1966.*

jet or beaten silver, and non-sparkly beads and brooches are best for daytime wear.'

By March 1964 Modern **Woman** Magazine was telling its readers that *'In most cases, big jewellery now looks out of place and delicate pieces and simple pearls come into their own again.'* Then, in 1965, plastics were hailed as the latest thing in jewellery, reflecting the fashion for bright,

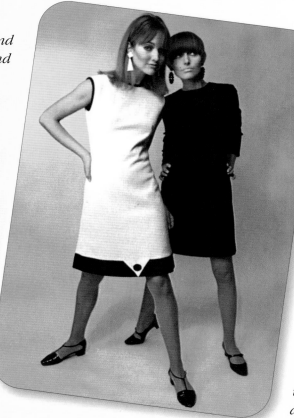

primary colours and Op Art designs, especially in the form of a target-like series of concentric circles, often in black and white, which could be seen on rings, earrings and brooches.

Vanity Fair in January 1966 advised those wishing to be in the latest style to *'pick star jewellery instead of the targets of last year. Stars can make cuff-links, rings, brooches and ear-rings, and can be white, yellow or silver.'*

Earrings, which had become one of

the most important items of jewellery with the advent of increasingly popular short hairstyles, were becoming bigger and more way out, and often made of brightly coloured plastics or precious metal. In September 1967 **Woman** magazine observed: *'…all's gold that glitters, as opposed to last year's silver. For the more way-out woman, latest ranges are in transparent Perspex plus the sharp shades. Try the whole co-ordinating set – earrings, bangle and ring.'*

Not jewellery as such, but paper flowers became all the rage in 1967, following the success of Scott McKenzie's hit record 'If You're Going to San Francisco' which advised that you should 'wear some flowers in your hair'. **Woman** magazine in May noted that *'it's questionable whether given the cash, today's teenager would cover herself in diamonds. She's much too stuck on flowers. Seen the paper ones you stick on your skin, pin in your hair, clip on your clothes? They have adhesive where real flowers have stems, are produced by Something Special, the two-girl firm. Pack of six, colour-assorted, costs 3s including postage.'* The magazine also gave instructions for a DIY version for wearing in your hair: *'Cut out petal shapes from 2in. squares of folded tissue paper. Pinch petals at base to form a flower shape. (Use about 30). Wind cotton tightly round base to secure. Sew on to a hairgrip.'*

With the arrival of the hippy look, more

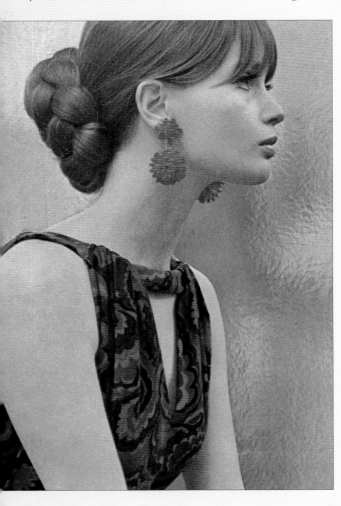

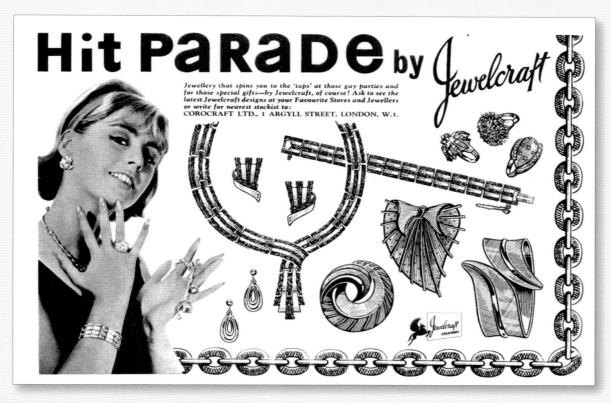

Hit PaRaDe by Jewelcraft

Jewellery that spins you to the 'tops' at those gay parties and for those special gifts—by Jewelcraft, of course! Ask to see the latest Jewelcraft designs at your Favourite Stores and Jewellers or write for nearest stockist to: COROCRAFT LTD., 1 ARGYLL STREET, LONDON, W.1.

Left *The words show it's the start of the 'swinging' era, but the jewellery-style hasn't quite caught up. October 1963.*

Below right *The hippy movement brought chunky ethni-stylec beads and rings to the fore.*

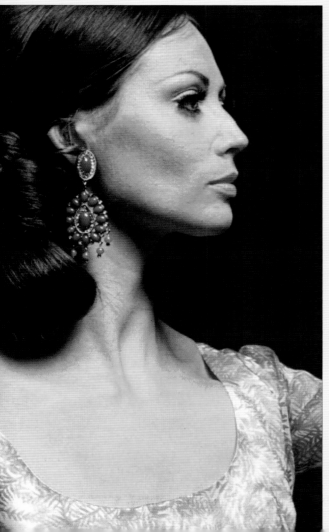

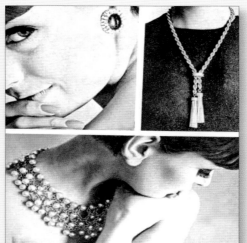

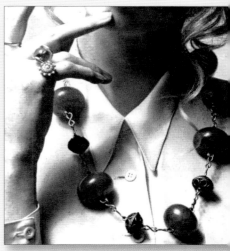

jewellery than ever was worn. One of the most common items was a small 'peace bell' hung around the neck, usually on a leather thong. These were replaced by Eastern-looking beads, and similar bangles and bracelets on the wrists, while on the fingers it became fashionable to wear several rings, often hand-made in silver. The outfit might well be finished with droopy earrings, which had been fashionable for some time, but now they were likely to be fashioned in an Indian-style.

Above left *Three examples of costume jewellery, from 1963.*

Far left *Indian-style pendant earrings were all the rage in the late sixties.*

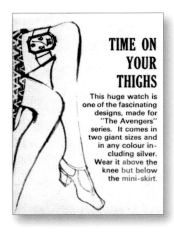

TIME ON YOUR THIGHS

This huge watch is one of the fascinating designs, made for "The Avengers" series. It comes in two giant sizes and in any colour including silver. Wear it above the knee but below the mini-skirt.

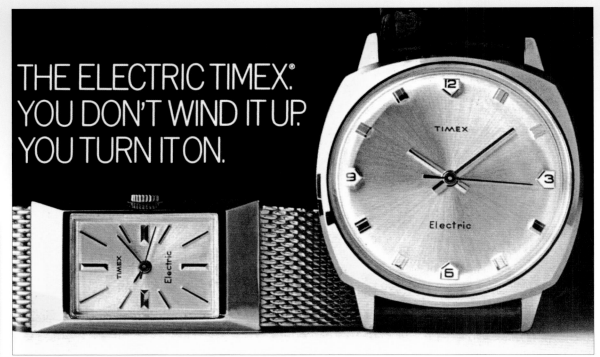

THE ELECTRIC TIMEX.®
YOU DON'T WIND IT UP.
YOU TURN IT ON.

Watches

As with most other items of clothing, the first few years of the 1960s saw little change in the appearance of wristwatches. For men, circular watches on leather wristbands were now almost universal, the most modern styles being slim, with a small window, usually on the right-hand side of the dial, showing the date. These soon dropped out of favour as, unless the month had thirty-one days, the watch had to be wound forward by twenty-four hours to set the date right when the month changed. The February/March changeover caused even more of a nuisance.

Women's watches were far more varied, with jewelled, usually diamanté, dress versions available for evening wear. The

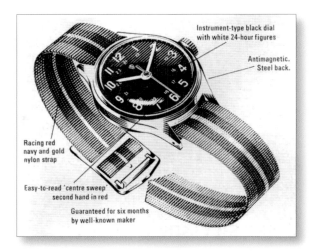

Instrument-type black dial with white 24-hour figures

Antimagnetic. Steel back.

Racing red navy and gold nylon strap

Easy-to-read 'centre sweep' second hand in red

Guaranteed for six months by well-known maker

faces were normally round, but square, oblong and shield-shaped were also available. Straps were either made of metal, leather or twisted cord.

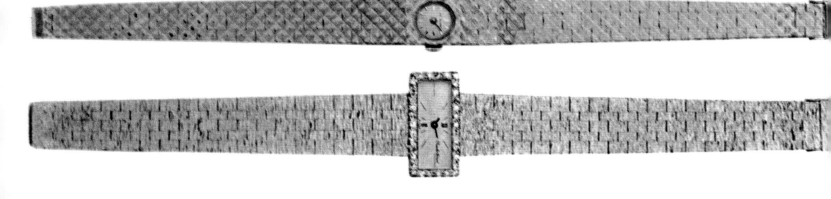

With the onset of the mid-decade swinging era, women's watches especially shook off the traditional style. To accentuate the little-girl look, men's watches were often worn, and these were later replaced by specially made large watches.

Watches were too expensive for most women to keep replacing them – a far cheaper alternative was a change of strap. Suede straps were the thing for a while, as were nylon straps in bright colours, often

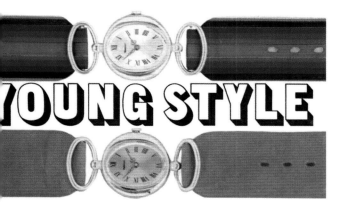

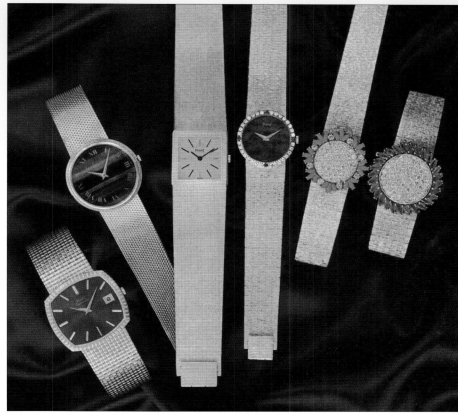

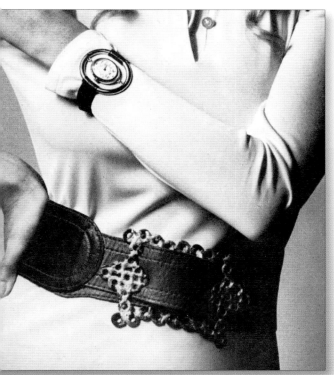

striped lengthways. Made in one piece, they could be changed in seconds to match your outfit. These were popular with both men and women.

In September 1967 **Woman** magazine announced: *'Watches – big time. Numbers appear either in Roman or bold figures. Autumn tickers have large circular or square faces with wide black suede or patent straps.'*

The latest innovations were the self-winding watch, which wound the spring by means of a weighted rotor activated by the movements of the wearer's arm, and the battery-powered electric watch which supplanted it and eventually became the norm. Another fashionable alternative for women was the pendant watch.

The end of the decade saw a revival of the jewelled dress-watch. Hippies on the other hand rarely wore watches at all.

Time-killers love this bold-faced suede-strapped timepiece; £4 19s. 6d. at Civil Service Stores.

Above *Not all jewellery was cheap and cheerful. These watches are in 18ct. gold and ranged from £575 up to £960 in October 1969!*

Far left, top *Chunky women's watches, on large, bright straps, 1968.*

Lower far left *Chunky watches were still fashionable, April 1969.*

Left *In 1967, the fashion in women's watches was big and chunky, this from July.*

SCARVES

Right A heaband tied at the back of the head beneath the hair, 1966.

Men

Men's scarves have changed little over the last century. Any significant differences usually take the form of altered details, such as material, pattern and length. Men almost always wore scarves as a functional item in cold weather. In terms of how they were worn, three main styles were pretty constant: knotted at the front of the neck, choker-style; the single twist round the neck, usually with one end to the front and one to the rear; and the ultra-cold-weather style: crossed over the chest and worn inside the overcoat.

At the end of the 1960s, with the arrival of the romantic and hippy styles, scarves became more ornamental, and they were worn either flamboyantly round the neck or tied round the head Apache Indian-style.

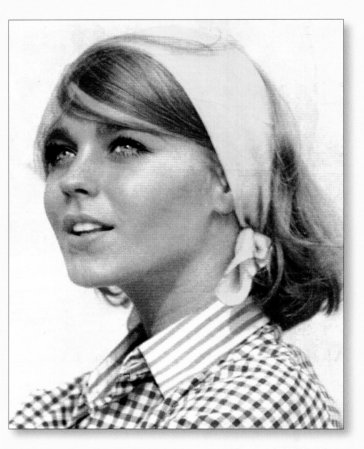

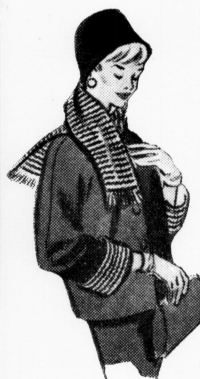

Above Scarf, November 1960, see instructions in text right.

Women

For women the scarf had always been a far more versatile garment. **Woman's Weekly** in November 1960 stated: *'A plain scarlet dress in wool jersey would be set off handsomely by a patterned, scarlet-bordered silk handkerchief. It could be worn as a scarf, a head-scarf, tied as a sash or simply falling out of a pocket.'*

The magazine went on to give instructions on how to *'give a collarless suit jacket a new throw-away scarf of plain rib. Knit a long straight strip, perhaps using a mixture of wool of the suit colour and* another colour. For example, with a black suit, use black and royal blue or black and brown wools.

How to attach it; sew the scarf to the back of the neck where the collar would have been; bring one end round to fall down in front, and pass the other over to the back. Three-quarter length sleeves could have cuffs of the same knit, turned back.'

A scarf could even be used like a sash to disguise a less-than-perfect body shape. In October 1961 **Housewife** magazine advised that *'The taller woman can wear gay scarves tied at one side to offset her slimness.'*

By far the most common use of the scarf was as a headscarf. The ends could be tied under the chin, but a more fashionable style was to tie it behind the neck. It soon became smart to wear a headscarf crossed under the chin and tied at the back of the neck, with the front of the scarf pushed back to allow the fringe to peep out. Many women used curlers to style their hair, and some would wear a headscarf to partially conceal the curlers.

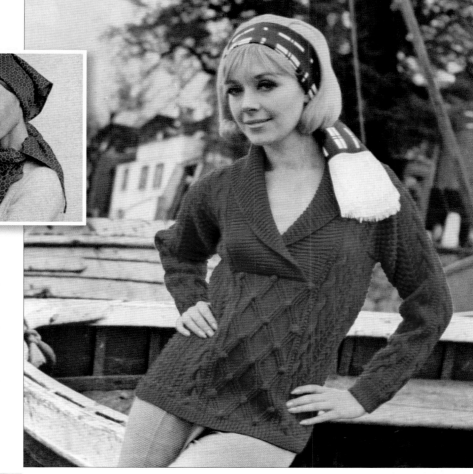

This fashion then changed, either to a much smaller headscarf tied under the chin which allowed both the fringe and the back of the hair to be seen, or even briefer, a scarf rolled into a thin strip and worn over the hair, Alice-band style, tied at the back of the neck.

By September 1967 **Woman** magazine was writing that the latest fashions in scarves were '*…more abstract and art nouveau, colours predominantly oranges and browns with classical paisley designs. Tie your scarf the French way, behind nape of*

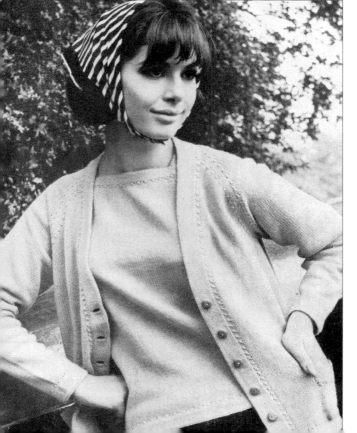

neck, giving fullness and width.'

In the late 1960s scarves and shawls became important fashion accessories: the romantic style was perfectly complemented by foulards – long, narrow lengths of wispy, floaty material, which normally had a printed design on them. These could be worn as an exotic turban, as a headscarf, or a bandana.

Shawls became popular, either worn around the shoulders in hippy peasant style, or wound around the hips and tied at the side. Another alternative was a long knitted muffler around the neck, sometimes so long that the ends reached the ground. **Woman's Realm** in August 1969 told its readers, '*Just tie a scarf around your head, neck or waist and you'll get a really bang-up-to-date top fashion look.*'

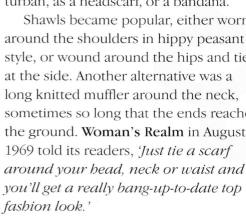

Above *Scarf worn as a headband, 1964.*

Inset above *Two scarves, worn in the fashionable peasant style, August 1969.*

Left *A small headscarf tied beneath the chin, 1964, allowing the fringe to peep out.*

WOMEN'S HAIR

1960

In the late 1950s and early 1960s hairstyles had begun to take a more natural, softer line. Mid- and full-length hair tended to be worn straight with the ends flicked up, while the higher hairstyle was a cross between a classical Greek look, and the youthful, almost cropped, gamine look. For special occasions, a trip to the hairdresser was the order of the day, but usually home perming and setting was the norm, and to this end women's magazines often gave instructions about how to create various hairstyles.

That year's **Boyfriend Annual** gave directions for up-to-the-minute hair styles: '*Carol's naturally fine hair is straight and thick and was already tapered in short lengths, so stylist Joan set it on twelve large*

rollers, finishing off the very short hair at the nape of the neck in pin curls. Six of the rollers from the crown of the head she rolled forward to get the effect of a heavy front fringe when brushed out, and six she rolled back to give fullness on the crown. When she back-brushed it the effect was like candyfloss, light and airy with an ice-pink sheen and a bouffant effect of sweeping fullness across the back of the head. The sides were soft and slightly bouffant, framing the face.'

Linda's fringe was swept across her forehead without pin or clip. The crown was set on large rollers – eight of them – rolling them back from her face. At the nape of the neck he made "barrel-curls", stuffing them with lumps of cotton wool to keep their shape under the drier. Her hair being swept two ways from an almost invisible parting, rising at the crown of the head to fall softly at the neck in an upturned sweep of deep curl.'

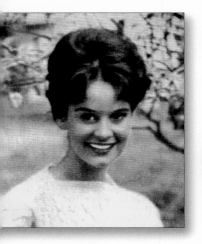

Above Long hair, January 1960.

Above The short, piled high style, January 1960.

Below Hairstyles in the early sixties were often of the birds'nest/beehive, high crowned style. This one could be anytime in the first half of the decade. Directions for setting the hair to achieve the hairstyle shown below.

Right and below Another hairstyle from the start of the sixties.

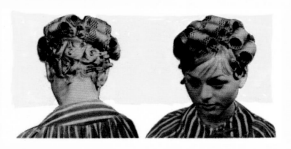

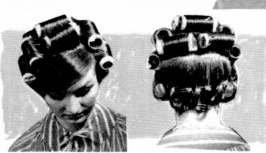

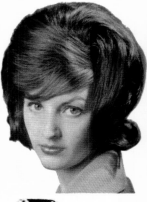

1961

Everyday hairstyles remained much the same, but fringes became more common.

In October **Housewife** magazine advised its readers how to get their hair back in shape after the summer holidays. The article gives some interesting insights into hair care at the time. *'The starting point is a new hairstyle, in conjunction with a good home treatment. Book an appointment with the best stylist you know; the sort of haircut you can get from him will be an investment; it will make home setting fun instead of a bore. Ask your hairdresser to do the most suitable cut for your type of hair. If you have fine hair he will club cut it: this means cutting straight across, in sections, which will make it more manageable and give the impression of greater body. If you have thick, coarse hair ask for a tapered cut (this is done by holding sections of hair at right angles to the head and slithering the scissors along it towards the roots). Tapering slightly thins the hair, giving wave and buoyancy to heavy, thick hair; then it is cut in layers to achieve a definite shape.'*

The article went on to recommend the best care, and cuts, for different types of hair. Fine and lanky hair should be shampooed every seven to ten days using a liquid shampoo and plenty of beer or wave-setting lotion to give body to the hair when setting. It should be brushed infrequently. For a polish, a piece of silk should be smoothed over the finished hairdo. For this type of hair, a short, springy cut was recommended, with a fairly strong permanent wave, curled right up to the roots of the hair.

For dry and coarse hair, once a month, before shampooing, a mixture of half castor and half olive oil was to be rubbed in thoroughly and left to soak in, under a hot, moist towel. It should be shampooed every ten days, using a cream shampoo, followed by a good conditioning cream, and a light perm was recommended.

With thick and greasy hair, a shampoo every three days was recommended, using a pine-based or medicated shampoo. If you had to use a brush, the advice was to touch the ends only, well away from the scalp, and to massage the scalp firmly with the fingertips. Layer cutting and thinning would make it easy to set at home and the use of beer kept the set in longer. If the hair was oily, a dry shampoo was recommended. This could be done in two ways: firstly by soaking pads of cotton wool in eau-de-cologne, then placing them between the bristles of a hairbrush and lightly brushing the oil out of the hair. Alternatively you could shake some dry shampoo into your hair, which would remove the grease as you brushed it out.

Over-curly hair needed regular warm oil treatments, and the application of conditioning cream after every shampoo. Frequent brushing was strongly recommended. Long hairstyles were not advised, unless the hair was wrapped in a chignon or French pleat after 'straightening'. This was described as permanent waving in reverse, and could be done in most hair salons.

Fine and dry hair required massaging the scalp with the fingertips each night and before shampooing. A warm olive and castor oil treatment was recommended every three weeks before washing with a cream shampoo. Women with fine and dry hair were advised to have shorter hair, well cut, with the very lightest of permanent waves set on large curlers.

What is most interesting about these instructions is how infrequently people were advised to wash their hair. Even as late as 1968 the **Boyfriend Annual** advised: *'Don't wash your hair more than once weekly.'*

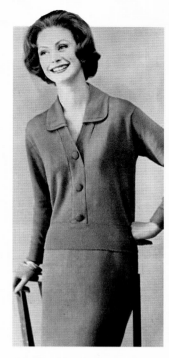

Above *The fashionable style tended to be medium long, and not overly lacquered. October 1961.*

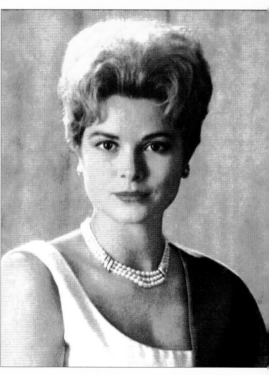

Above *Princess Grace of Monaco in May 1961 sporting the high look.*

1962

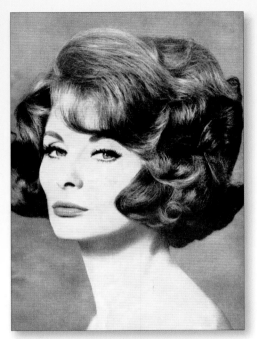

In Paris Yves Saint Laurent popularised an evening style where the hair was piled high in a towering chignon. Meanwhile **Woman's Journal** magazine asked top-notch London hairdressers to predict the coming season's hit hairstyles. The answer was *'still softly casual but with plenty of movement'.*

The illustration *(left)* shows one example, by Robert at Richard Henry, who *'plumps for the little mop cap coiffure for young devastation. Cropped for roundness and a little bit of height, it has a roaring Twenties headband peeping between "pouffe bangs" – deep fringes swinging across the forehead to join silky tendrils of hair slinking close down to the nape of the neck and tipping gently over the ears.'*

The magazine went on to give directions: *'Perming need be only very, very light, and healthy, shining hair is a "must" for this style to be a success. The shape depends entirely on good cutting – when the cut is right, all you need is a brush to restore the line.*

'Setting: Set sides and back with rollers and pin-curls as shown. Divide the front hair into a high parting and wind rollers away from the parting, towards the ears. Set immediate front section over one large roller to shape fringe.

'Comb-out: Brush hair through and through in the direction in which the rollers are set, coaxing it into soft, undulating waves with ends out-flicked to spice the silhouette. Mould hair at the nape of the neck close to the head.'

In May **Modern Woman** looked at that summer's styles: *'Simplicity is the keyword to summer hairstyles – the newest look shows a distinct trend towards softer styles with more of an upward sweep. Length? A little longer than we've been wearing it. Result? No more excessive back-combing and a hairdo that's easy to look after yourself.'*

Another style, the Beehive, would be one of the classics of the sixties. It combined the two styles which had come to

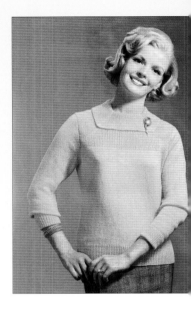

Above *April 1962*

dominate women's hair; the mid-length and the high on top. Interestingly this particular set of instructions came from an advert for Amami wave set, which included the lines; *'Today's hair fashions need a deep down set to hold them. A hairspray alone is not enough. That's why, after your shampoo, you must use Amami Wave Set first.'* Clearly, hair sprays were beginning to bite into the setting and permanent market.

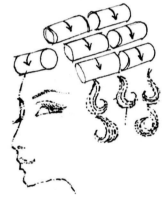

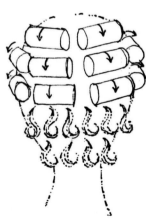

Above *Directions for setting the hair to achieve the hairstyle shown in the photo above.*

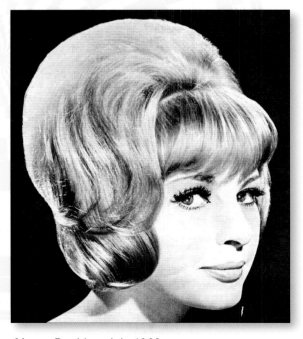

Above *Beehive, July 1962.*

1963

In January **Modern Woman** wrote that *'we'll wear short, short styles hugging close at the nape, with a single curl coming forward over each ear, during the early part of the year. Later in the summer we'll start growing our locks again and wearing them loose at the nape with crown hair coiled high on top. Watch out for more developments in the wig industry – they're getting cheaper and cheaper, harder and harder to distinguish from the real thing! I expect to see more colour shampoos.'*

In 1963 Vidal Sassoon created the 'Nancy Kwan' hairstyle, which the actress wore in the film *The Wild Affair*. In 1959 Sassoon had created the 'Shape', a layered cut with the hair swept forward from the crown to fall in points at the curve of the jaw. This became the basis for a series of angular hairstyles cut on a horizontal plane, based on the classic 'bob' of the 1920s and '30s. These geometric haircuts were severely cut, but once done they freed women from continually back-combing and teasing their hair into shape, and were lacquer-free which made them very low maintenance. The epitome of the style was the 'Five Point' cut, also known as the Mary Quant, because it had been seen first at her fashion show, and was worn by Quant herself.

Sassoon later described its effect: 'It was a radical change. People either loved or hated it. The Press gave us marvellous write-ups or shrieked with fury because we were trying to make women "ugly" or "like men".' Not everyone, of course, went for this severe style. **Woman's Weekly** that May gave instructions for a variation on the piled-high style.

'The ends were trimmed a little to stop breaking and the short front wisps were cut into a definite fringe. The hair was washed with a soapless shampoo and given a plastic setting lotion to add body, It was then set on medium-sized rollers – very large ones wouldn't give the necessary "bounce" to this

SLEEK CURVE   SOFT WAVE   FIRM WAVE   STRONG WAVE   CRISP CURL

fine hair. When it was dry, it brushed out into new fluffiness and was arranged in the beautifully shaped "pleat" style. Most amateurs, when trying to put their hair up, handle too much hair at once. The professional hairdresser sections off the hair and handles one piece at a time (diagram 1). First the back hair was arranged into a pleat, then the two side sections were brushed back over the ears and pinned on top of the pleat. Then the top hair was swirled around to form the pretty bun which finished off the top of the pleat (2). Finally, the fringe was arranged in position – this could be brushed to one side or worn down as shown. Each strand of hair was lightly back-brushed with a soft bristle brush to give it a thicker appearance before being pinned into position.'

Above A good range of fashionable styles from January 1963.

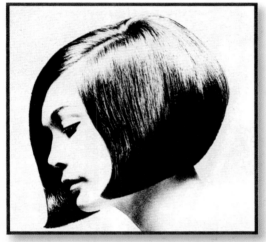

Above The 'Nancy Kwan' cut, by Vidal Sassoon.

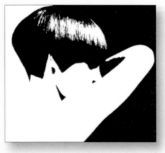

Left The 'Five point' cut, by Vidal Sassoon, a style made famous by Mary Quant.

Below Instructions for achieving the piled-high look, May 1963.

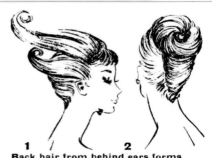 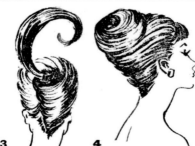

1   2   Back hair from behind ears forms lower pleat, side pieces pinned back. Top hair forms top swirl.

3   4   For extra height a false switch can be added and swirled round to give a " bun " effect.

1964

Many older women were still wearing the longer, back-combed, flicked-up hairstyles which were the direct descendants of the

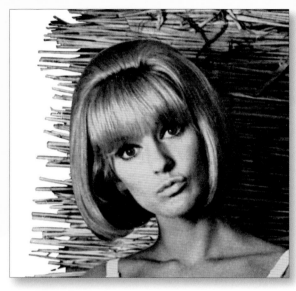

Right *Medium length, backcombed hairstyle, very typical of the period, September 1964.*

Far right *Egyptian-style, Summer 1964 – 'Cleopatra' had been the previous year's smash hit film, making all things with an ancient Egyptian feel fashionable.*

1950s style, but this was slowly changing. For younger women the most common style remained a more rigid version of the same cut, but with a fringe, and with the side and back hair turning inwards.

Boyfriend Annual that summer carried an article on 'Swingy new hair', and if the headline alone doesn't alert you, the style of the article leaves the reader in no doubt that the Swinging 1960s have really arrived.

'If you want to get ahead, get a new hairstyle – and get it fast! Don't cling to back-combing and beehives. Buy a false piece of hair made up into a pleat, a mesh, twist-band, or switch. Way-out chicks could try the "falsies" in contrasting colours for a dazzling effect. But be very careful, for these switches used the wrong way can make you "way-out" in both senses of the word!

'The fashion makers have been putting their heads together to give you girls a swingy new hair-line for winter. And they've agreed on two things:
1. The sleeker, tailored look is on its way in.
2. Short hair is a must – but you could stretch it to medium if you hanker after long looks.

Above *The 'Demure' style, Summer 1964... It softly flicks up at the ends and comes forward on to the face in kiss-curls. The full fringe is gently swept to one side. On top, a piece of false hair, which has been set to fit into her own hair, is attached. Finish with a narrow velvet ribbon tied in a bow.*

'Try and make your hairstyle reflect your personality. It's not much good stay-at-home tele-types going for high, exaggerated hairdos. Take a look at our girls – they'll give you an idea how to boost your morale in the cold days ahead. Sally's quiet. She prefers a good book to living it up at the local palais. Her tastes are simple, but she sometimes likes to cut a dash on a "heavy" date.

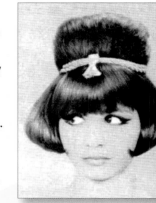

'Anne's lively. She reads pop magazines like **Boyfriend***, goes to the cinema twice a week and is game for any zany fashions. She's so with-it – she's way ahead! Ideal for her is the "Miss Cleo" It's high, wide and handsome! The full fringe and bouffant sides are balanced by height on top. The bun bit is her own hair, but if yours isn't long enough, buy a falsie and attach it. Get the real Cleo effect by tying a double piece of cord round the top-knot. And, of course, to top this Cleo look, the make-up must be matching too. We don't mean for you to go the whole hog with the eyes, but, as you can see on our model, slightly exaggerated eye-lines help to enhance the charming hairstyle.'*

Modern Woman in October 1964 gave advice on the latest hair styles. *'No more wind-tossed hair or shiny complexions; your hair has a neater look, and is arranged in a smooth shining cap or the more elaborate sophisticated styles with a hint of the hours that used to be spent on coiffure in the olden days, but not since switches came into fashion.*

'Autumn hairstyles are often dictated by the new hat fashion'. For those who want to wear the latest in hats, *'As well as the bathing cap there are small berets and helmets perched well forward on the brow. Hair is cut to the minimum to fit underneath.'*

1965

The **Boyfriend Annual** that year gave a resumé of the latest styles. *'Now that birds' nests and busbies are fading out, sleekness is an absolute must. Slightly longer hair is more fashionable, but this doesn't mean that you should let it straggle down your neck. Long locks need just as good a cut as short ones. If your hair is over curly, then it's best not to grow it. A short bob will be much easier to keep tidy than a long one which only looks good immediately after it's been set.*

'Fringes enjoyed a long popularity, but they are disappearing. Here you must make your own decision. *Very high foreheads need a few fronds on them. Narrow foreheads appear to be wider when the hair is swept right off over to one side. During the past year there has been a big rebellion against too vigorous back-combing and lacquer.'*

The annual recommended *'a pin curl set – the pin curls are upright, smothered in setting lotion and each one is kept in place with a clip.'* For those who want height it recommended a process called "throwing". *'Pieces of hair are casually flicked with the brush instead of being brushed right down to the roots, leaving a tangled mess beneath a smooth top.'*

Rave magazine told its readers in May that *'There are two "In" hairstyles. Very curly or very straight. The loose, floppy curls Pet Clark sports these days – they're In. If you don't go for this style, my tip: go right to the other extreme and wear your hair long and straight.'*

At the end of October, **Woman** magazine provided suggestions for parties: *'Hair-dos in-a-trice. A fun plait for parties from a skein of chunky wool. Anchor with grips, wear loose or coiled into a chignon. Prettier still: stud with flowers for festive look. Pin two giant swansdown powder puffs – one green, one beige – at nape.'*

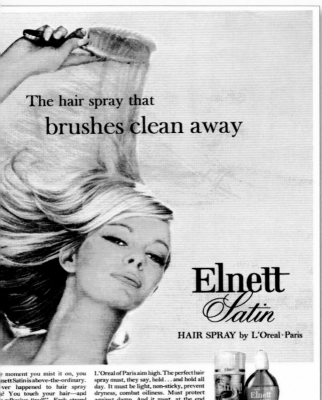
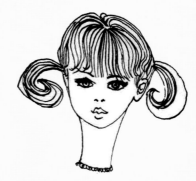

Left *Very up-to-date hairstyle and make-up, 1965.*

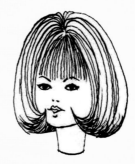

Above *The latest styles of 1965.*

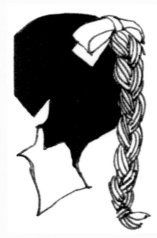

Above and below left *Party hair, from Woman magazine, October 1965.*

Far left *The latest styles needed control, yet with a natural look – hair spray, July 1965.*

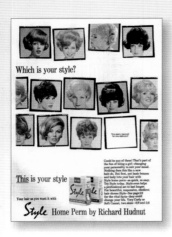

Above A wide range of hairstyles from May 1966.

1966

While beehives and birds' nests were still to be seen, they were certainly less fashionable, while the trend for short hair remained, but cut in a wide range of styles. This shorter style looked very smart on older women, and many of them were happy to adopt it as the general fashion for a younger look really began to take hold. Low maintenance was important; busy working women and housewives needed to be able to do their everyday hair quickly and easily, while at the same time it had to be simply converted into a stylish evening hairstyle.

Woman magazine in September gave instructions for *'three vivacious styles for short hair all from one set. Take your choice of two styles for day and an elegant adaptation for evening wear. The hair should be professionally cut – the crown hair is four inches long, graduating to one inch at the nape. The sides are tapered from the fringe to ear tips, and the fringe is four inches long.*

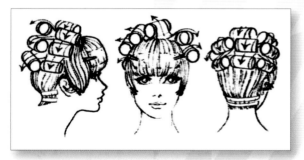

'The hair is wound on to medium rollers, and the fringe is combed forward over a thick strip of cotton wool, secured at each side with a clip. Comb the side hair smoothly in front of each ear, curving the ends back and clipping in position. The lower back hair is combed straight and secured on the neck with sticky tape.'

'Brush hair around head, sweeping front hair and fringe to the right. The left side is combed in front of ear in direction of set. Brush the nape hair flat on to neck. Now back-comb the top crown hair for height and smooth it back. The right side is

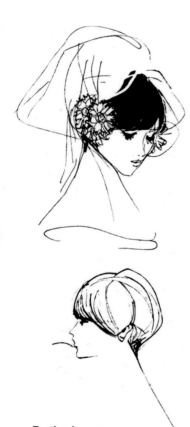

Both above
January 1966, how to wear the 'space age crop' for a bride.

brushed back from the face and then forward with back hair; back-comb the ends a little to achieve a fan shape. The lower right side hair is combed on to cheek. Lift crown and right side with a hairpin and secure with spray (photo right, above).'

Alternatively, 'Brush hair through firmly in direction of set, so that the fringe is taken on to the brow and the sides curve gently in front of ears. The nape hair is combed flat on neck. Back-comb the crown hair and smooth it sleekly around head to merge with the rest of hair. Lift crown and sides for height and width. Set the style lightly with spray (photo above right).

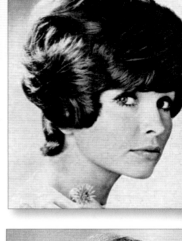

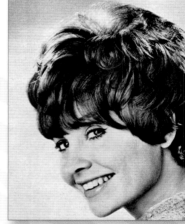

The evening adaptation *(photo lower right)* was achieved as follows: 'Brush fringe on to brow and comb curved sidepieces through in direction of set. Brush the nape hair flat on neck. Back-comb crown hair one section at a time, smoothing the sections one by one and arranging them around the crown in soft feathers. Bring front crown hair forward towards the fringe. Lift crown and sides with a hairpin for height and width and set lightly with spray to help keep the shape.'

In January **Vanity Fair** magazine gave tips for styling a bride's hair: '...*her heavy fringe is parted, clipped back under demure clusters of giant white daisies. Going away, she shakes back into a space age crop.'*

1967

The May issue of **Woman** magazine gave tips for styling your own hair: *'The right equipment [is] essential – not getting it together in bits and pieces but acquiring it all from the start: rollers in suitable sizes plus pins and clips for flat curls, a circular bristle brush, tail comb, as well as setting lotion, spray, a good conditioner and lots of patience.'*

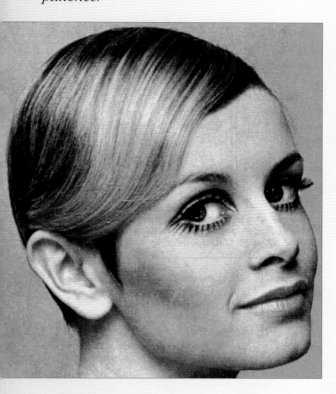

Some women continued to wear their hair short, but the overall fashion was for longer hair. Hair was grown to at least shoulder length, sometimes permed, or if naturally wavy, allowed to fall in a tangle of curls. For those with short hair, a hairpiece or a wig was a good way of faking it. *'Good-looking wigs can now be bought for 10 guineas (the Carmen range comes in thirty blended hair colours). Like fake pieces, wigs should be kept wound up in rollers, when not being worn. It's easiest to slip out the rollers, brush through, and finally comb through when on the head.'*

Woman magazine advised its readers: *'Switch to plaits. Put fun into a really*

shortie hairdo with a perky pair of plaits. Made from two plaited Dynel switches, attached to a plastic alice band and daisy-trimmed; eye-catching for any party. Secret is to plait as tightly as possible so they will hold their shape and to anchor plait ends with an elastic band and slip on to the alice band. Cover the elastic band with a fake, or – for one evening only – a real flower.' Alternatively, *'short, straight Twiggy-length hair is dressed-up for dates with pop-on ringlets.'*

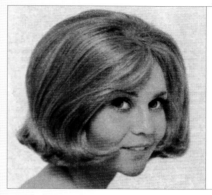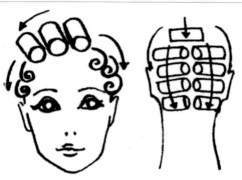

Woman magazine in September gave directions for a longer style (shown above): *'Length: Club cut to jaw length or longer. Brush through hair. Back-brush lightly at roots working from a point just left of forehead, comb down sides. Sweep right side in curve over forehead. Press in wave with side of hand, combing ends upward over hand and on to cheek. Comb down left side, flipping ends under. Smooth crown hair back and comb sleekly into nape.'*

They also gave instructions for the more bubbly style (shown right): *'Length: Six to eight inches on crown; three to four inches at sides. Brush through hair. Comb down fringe and side sections, coaxing hair into loose curls with tailcomb. Back-brush hair lightly all over crown. Then working from central point divide hair into small sections and comb ends in curls round crown. Work over back of head in the same way.'*

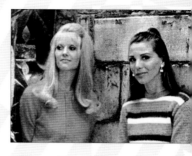

Above Two fashionable longer styles from September 1967.

Far left Most styles were longer, but you could still get away with the Twiggy-style short crop.

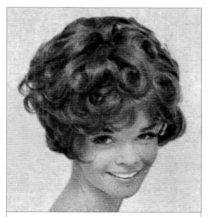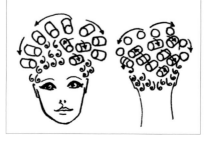

1968

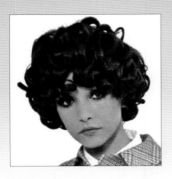

Above The 'Moppet look', modeled by Cathee Dahman, January 1968.

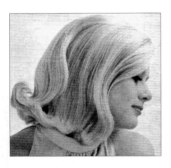

Above A romantic effect was the aim in 1968.

Far right The long page boy cut for the more confidently daring.

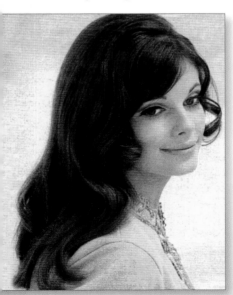

Above Very long hair was also very much in fashion.

One of the more fashionable styles was called 'the Moppet look'. The hair style was described by **Honey** magazine as *'curly, of course, short sweet and Shirley Temple, or a romantic ruffle of ringlets.'* **Woman** showed how to achieve the look in the January issue.

'Curls vary from tight corkscrews to a Harpo Marx (deliberately frizzed) halo. Happy medium: loose, roll-mop curls, as in this style.

'Unless hair is naturally curly, a light body perm may be needed to make curls last. Short hair if it's six inches or less in length – will gain a tight, even longer-lasting curl if set on perm rollers (twenty rollers for a full set will do the trick). When the hair is dry, brush through well, sweeping all hair upwards and away from face. Then, starting from crown, wind chunky sections of hair round finger to make loose roll-curls. Flick side hair towards face, up at nape. Press gently with palms to flatten. With a hairpin separate curls to give an over-all bubbly look.'

Apart from this, long hair was most certainly in fashion, worn in a flowing, romantic style, slightly raised in the crown and then allowed to fall loose onto the shoulders. In practice this style meant that the hair would fall forward onto the face, especially when the woman was leaning forward. This encouraged a habit of shaking or tossing the head back to clear the face and eyes, a gesture which became very common, as did the practice of hooking hair over and behind the ears while reading, writing or performing some similar activity. Once again, **Woman** showed how to achieve the style. *'Corkscrew-ringlets just at cheek level give a bang-up-to-the-minute look, make a pretty disguise for an out-growing fringe.*

'Set hair over medium-size rollers wound towards the back. Divide shorter side hair into two sections and comb into flat pin curls. When dry, remove rollers and brush all hair back from forehead. Back-brush lightly at crown and allow hair to fall naturally to shoulders. Remove pin curls. Wind strands of hair round tail-comb, draw tail downwards to form ringlets of hair. Spray to hold. For added flick-ups or to straighten too wavy hair, direct dryer to hair and keep combing.'

They also suggested a style for older women: *'Mid-length hair has been ousted by short curly cuts and the perennial long, flowing manes. But if you're thirty-plus or are growing your hair, a hint of wave adds a trendy touch.*

'Set all hair on medium rollers wound towards the back. For a quick set use water-heated rollers for ten minutes. Remove rollers and spray curls lightly before brushing out (this gives added body, makes mid-length hair that is much easier to manage). Brush hair down from short parting on left, flicking brush bristles upwards at hair tips to form casual curls. Place a grip at cheekbone level on right side. With tail comb gently lift hair at crown then swirl one section from back crown to right, pin to secure. Spray lightly. Remove holding grip.'

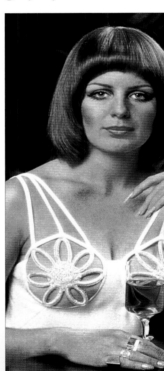

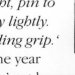

Later in the year the 'page-boy' cut became popular. The hair was styled flat and close to the head, with the sides shaped and falling to the nape of the neck. It was so called because the style resembled the coiffure worn by pages in medieval pictures.

1969

The simple yet innovative styles of the mid-1960s had now virtually disappeared. Popular lengths of hair were around the jawline, or shoulder length plus. Long hair was often styled elaborately for more formal occasions, while variations on the page-boy and the bob were still seen.

Woman's Realm recommended hairstyles for various facial types: *'For a round face*

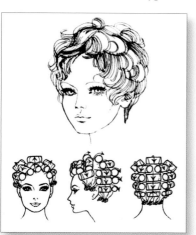

(see left) – chubby cheeks and a plumpish rounded jawline. Do keep hair close and fairly flat at the sides, high at the crown. This will lengthen and slim your face-shape.

'Don't let hair grow below ear-tip level (unless you're going to brush it back into a French pleat) or wear your hair sleek to your head with a centre parting. This will only accentuate roundness.

'Use medium-size rollers (if hair is more than four inches at crown); small-size rollers if hair is shorter. Pin at forehead, sides and back as shown in sketches.

'Brush through hair away from the face, gently back-brush all over except for nape and sides. Smooth nape hair into place. With tail end of comb, tease side and forehead curls forward. Press side curls flat with the palms of your hands and then surface-smooth back-brushed hair into flattering forward-flicking and overlapping curls and waves. Then spray the hair to hold the set in place.'

'For a heart-shaped face (see above right) – broad brow, definite bone structure, with well-formed high cheekbones, and a smallish chin. Do wear your hair in ripple waves to the shoulders, with height at the

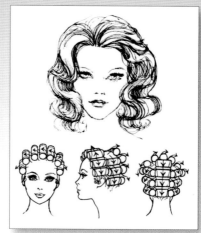

forehead (no parting) to accentuate face-shape. Or side hair can be pinned behind ears to show off high cheekbones and a pert chin. Don't wear hair with a centre or high parting so that a fall of hair hides your face-shape. Don't wear a fringe, you'll hide that favoured widow's peak effect.

'Use large-sized rollers, pin side curls as shown.

'Brush all hair back from face. Remove rollers, leave pin-curls in place. Brush hair back from face. Back-brush crown and front. Smooth over. Make tiny off-centre parting with tail end of comb to divide front hair slightly; smooth with hand. Remove pin-curls. To get waves at sides and back, press side of hand to form hollow, pushing bottom hair up to hand and then moving it down to the tips of hair. Use a little light hairspray to hold in place.'

'For a square face (see right) – a medium or low forehead, with a jutting jawline. Do keep hair at medium-length; with ends feathered or fluted just above the jawline to soften and minimise the square effect. Don't wear hair in a severe or geometric cut, close to the face or pulled back to reveal jawline. Don't wear a full fringe – it will only shorten your face and just make it appear more square-shaped. Use medium-sized rollers except for two small ones at the nape.

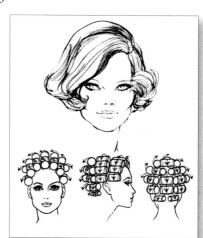

'Brush hair down from full (i.e., forehead to crown) side parting at left. Back-brush lightly at crown and more firmly at roots of back and side hair. With brush bristle-tips gently smooth over hair on right of parting, flicking ends under then slightly forward to checks. Again with a brush, smooth down the hair on left of parting, this time flicking curls upwards to about eyebrow level. Keep the back hair smooth and gently curled under. Spray to hold set.'

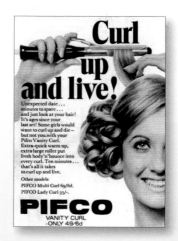

Above The latest curly look meant that curling tongs became very popular.

MEN'S HAIR

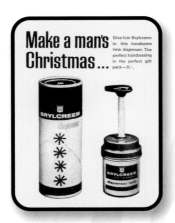

Above *December 1964, for the young, hairdressing meant Brylcreem.*

At the start of the decade men's hairstyles were very much the same as they had been for the last twenty years – basically the short back and sides. A visit to the barbers was simple; all you had to decide was how much you wanted off, and whether you wanted 'anything for the weekend'. As the name suggests, hair was cut short around the sides and back, but left long on the top. This might be very long, and unruly hair was kept in check with hairdressing, most popularly Brylcreem. The main problem with the short back and sides was that it made even teenagers look middle-aged, and with the new trend towards a youthful look, its days were numbered.

The alternative had been the American crew-cut. This developed into the continental-style 'crop' or 'French crop'; it was less severe than the crew-cut, and went perfectly with the fashionable slimline look in suits and ties.

It is difficult to imagine the shock caused by the Beatles' hairstyles when they and other unconventional new bands burst onto the music scene in 1962. Compared with the short back and sides, the crew-cut and the crop, their hair was positively long with its

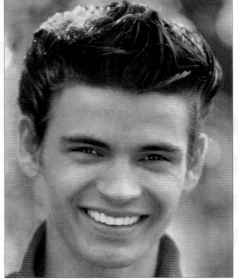

Above left *Don Everly, 1961, plenty of dressing, but the style still concentrates on the top.*

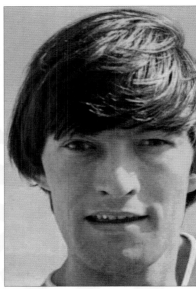

Above right *Dave Berry, 1966, and hair is beginning to creep down the back and sides.*

fringe cut straight across the forehead, and sides which covered the ears. It seemed quite outrageous at the time. This hairstyle led to the Americans dubbing them 'moptops'.

Their look became all the rage – thousands of young men tried to copy their clothes and hair, causing many an argument with their parents. Even if they won, hair takes time to grow, so the popular press carried adverts for 'Beatle wigs', most of which really did make you look as if you were wearing a black mop on your head.

The Mods were influenced by Italian styling; they took the sleek Italian cut and made it their own. The resulting hairstyle was the 'Mod' crop, the most severe cut being the half-inch, with a razored parting. **Rave** magazine in May 1965 advised their

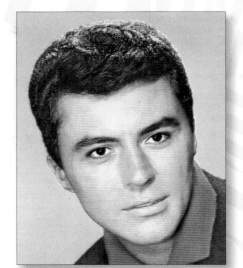

Above *James Darren, 1961, with a very Italian looking crop.*

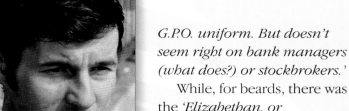

readers that *'For boys who want 'In' heads. Long hair is right out. Doomy. Also out is the close-cropped, nearly shaved style. Hair must be crisp and short – but still thick enough to be styled; and down the neck but not thick there. Ace examples are Steve McQueen, Rick and Sandy, and RSG's own Dave Goldsmith.'* (RSG was the smash-hit TV show **Ready Steady Go**).

Now there were genuine choices for the young and fashionable: to have your hair cut short into a crop like the Mods and stars such as Gene Pitney, or to let it grow long like the Rockers or the Rolling Stones, who had taken over from the Beatles as hate-figures for those who thought long hair effeminate.

Over the next few years, the Mod movement began to fracture into the hard Mods, who would develop into the skinheads, and the peacock Mods, who went with the more hippy-influenced psychedelic look. Hair was grown to cover the collar if possible. Once again, for those who could not wait, or more especially for those whose jobs meant that having long hair was not an option, or for those losing their hair, wigs were available in the latest styles.

Hair continued to be worn longer, and might be kept in place by a beaded headband. Beards and moustaches became very popular, and sideburns were grown to the bottom of the ear or longer. In June 1968 **Men Only** reported that *'We live in hairy times. Only the other day a panel of TV pundits, pronouncing on the chief characteristic of British society in the late twentieth century, discarded promiscuity, the swings to drugs, pop music, frozen foods and voted for 'hairiness'.'*

The article went on to look at styles of moustaches that were popular, including *'The Viva Zapata, or Mexican bandido. A relative newcomer, but already top of the pops. Suits pop stars and Mexican bandits, and should be worn with at least one of the following: guitar, embroidered Afghan jacket, or bandillero. No real reason why eccentric postman shouldn't wear it with*

G.P.O. uniform. But doesn't seem right on bank managers (what does?) or stockbrokers.'

While, for beards, there was the *'Elizabethan, or Mephistophelean. This handsome beard looks best with pointed eyebrows, and at least one wearer advises that for full effect, horns and a tail should also be worn. All right for writers and artists but too conspiratorial for politicians, and dangerous for parsons. When worn with shoulder length hair, a small moustache, and melancholy expression this style is more properly known as The Charlie Boy, after King Charles I, who had quite a lot to be melancholy about. The Charlie Boy has geographical limitations, being well thought of in the King's Road, but in bad taste in Scotland and the House of Commons.'*

Left George McClean, Dundee footballer, the style is short on top, but the sideburns give it away as March 1969.

Below For men whose hair refused to keep pace with the 1960's fashion for long flowing-locks, a range of male wigs were designed by 'Teasy Weasy' that retailed at about twelve guineas.

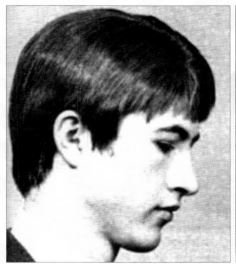
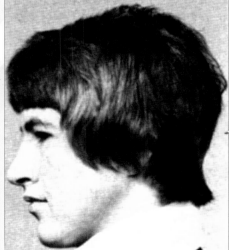
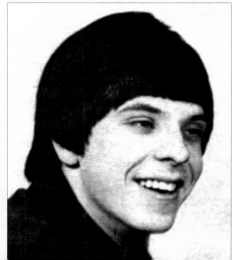
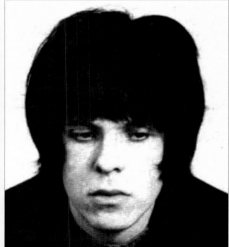

THE FIGURE

Men

In the past, a man's figure had been far less important to him than was the case with women. Now all that changed. Along with the long, slim-cut suit and tight trousers, the ideal figure for men was slim, and the young look prevailed.

Above Charles Atlas advert, April 1964.

Cute, baby-faced pop stars, such as Paul McCartney or Davy Jones of the Monkees were the new icons as the rugged look of the 1950s lost favour. Taken with the fashion for longer hair, this led to complaints from irate establishment types that it was impossible to tell boys from girls.

Teenage boys joined their sisters on diets. **Men Only** in April 1968 declared somewhat hopefully that *'The skinny-figure fad, which led to the emergence of Twiggy and the English Boy Look among male models, has reached almost an ultimate.'*

Women

The Perfect Figure

Right The 'sporty' figure, more rounded and natural looking than those of the forties and fifties. April 1968.

In February 1968 **Men Only** magazine stated *'Attractiveness is not a standard, neither is beauty. A look at the fat-bottomed femmes fatales of the early twentieth century, the slim-hipped big-busted beauties who replaced them in the 'thirties and 'forties, and the breastless wonders who rule the roosters nowadays, proves that time marches on. The pounds of bosom required to be a beauty twenty years ago now add up to only a handful of coppers. Both genders emphasised their particular sex by use of the chest line. More recently we have both been emphasising our sex (or our sexiness) by way of the leg line.'*

The overall theme that every age has its ideal figure and face is absolutely correct, while the lament about the then-fashionable look encapsulated the feelings of an older generation of men who yearned for the 'good old days' when the fashionable female look was for ample-bosomed beauties whose charms were emphasised by pointed bras. In fact, as can be seen from a cursory look at photos of women at the time, the flat chests which they complained of were in reality quite rare.

The fashion for a youthful look changed the ample figures of the 1950s; curves

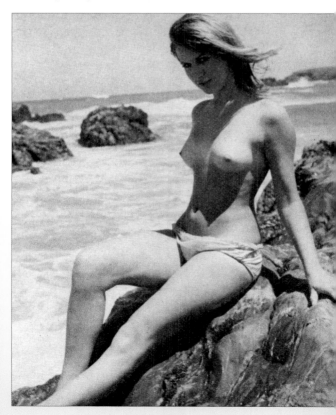

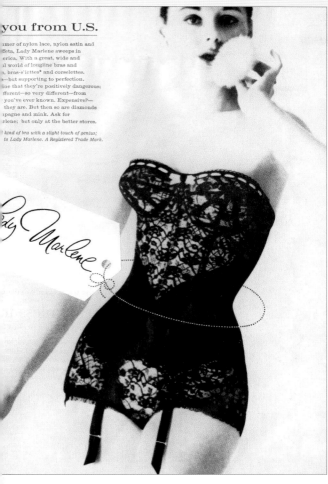

you from U.S.

...mer of nylon lace, nylon satin and
...feta, Lady Marlene sweeps in
...erica. With a great, wide and
...l world of longline bras and
..., bras-s'lettes' and corselettes.
...—but supporting to perfection.
...ine that they're positively dangerous;
...fferent—so very different—from
... you've ever known. Expensive?—
...they are. But then so are diamonds
...pagne and mink. Ask for
...rlene; but only at the better stores.

... kind of bra with a slight touch of genius;
... to Lady Marlene. A Registered Trade Mark.

became far softer, chests smaller and, as
hemlines rose, legs longer. **Woman**
magazine informed its readers in July 1962
that *'Long, lissom legs are every girl's ideal,
but petite and in-between ones can be just
as attractive. Length adds grace but what
really matters is shape and outline that
peters down from firmly-rounded thighs to
slimly-moulded ankles.'*

The magazine's advice was to stand
before a full-length mirror. *'Kick off your
shoes and face your reflection with feet
together and a strong resolve not to cheat.
Now watch where your legs meet. Ideally,
it's at four points – thighs, knees, calves and
ankles, with only a glimmer of light
showing between calves and ankles. If you
can grip a penny at each of those points, the
chances are your legs are in good shape
and a little regular care will keep them that
way. But if gaps and bulges mar the line,*

you need to get down to some shaping up.'

Men Only, however, continued its
campaign, writing in April 1968: *'The mini is
giving way to the maxi only because the
mini can get no minnier. Is it not logical
that there will be a fashionable swing back
to chests and breasts and hips and buttocks
now that the thinny can get no thinnier?'*
And again in November 1969: *'Since the war,
models and mannequins have got steadily
skinnier until one begins to wonder if one
is looking at a woman or a roll of
linoleum.'* They would have been heartened
to read **Woman** magazine in January 1968
declare that *'What is well beyond dispute is
that curves are making a comeback.'*

Dressing For Your Shape

As **Woman's Weekly** magazine pointed out
in October 1969: *'Your figure depends to a
certain extent on your individual build. If,
for instance, nature gave you narrow
shoulders, a small bust and wide hips, or
broad shoulders, a small waist and slim
hips, you could not alter your basic shape.'*
Magazines regularly made suggestions for
making the most of your particular figure. As
the **Boyfriend Annual** of 1961 put it: *'In
these days of high fashion off-the-peg there's
not the slightest need for any girl to be an
unfashionable ugly duckling. Fat or
thin, short or like a beanpole, if she
is clever she will find clothes that
make her the most elegant swan.'*

It went on to give tips for various
figures, including *'the small girl'* (5
feet 2 inches and under): *'Beware of
long jackets – they make you look as
if you're growing out of the ground.
But keep your skirts short – long
skirts won't make you look taller. Let
a long expanse of leg do that for
you. Short girls really look much better in
dresses than in suits. If you're small don't
have too many frills and furbelows – your
little self will get completely lost in all that
drapery. Don't wear lots of different colours*

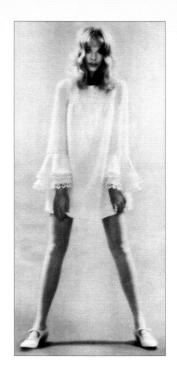

Left The dominance of
white in foundations and
underwear is being
challenged by US
manufacturers, June 1961.

Above The sixties' look –
long colt-like legs, an
unpronounced chest and
big eyes. January 1968.

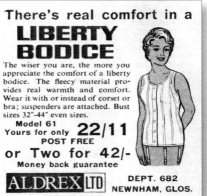

There's real comfort in a

LIBERTY BODICE

The wiser you are, the more you
appreciate the comfort of a liberty
bodice. The fleecy material pro-
vides real warmth and comfort.
Wear it with or instead of corset or
bra; suspenders are attached. Bust
sizes 32"-44" even sizes.

Model 61
Yours for only **22/11**
POST FREE
or **Two for 42/-**
Money back guarantee

ALDREX LTD   DEPT. 682
NEWNHAM, GLOS.

Above Even by February
1968, the Liberty bodice
was still a favourite.

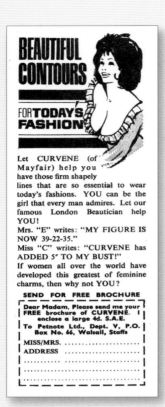

Above Advert from January 1966.

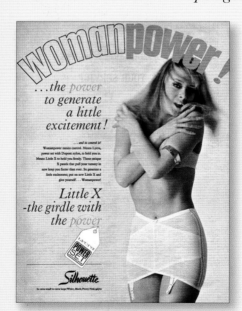

Far right Chart from September 1963, giving the number of calories required to 'maintain' your weight.

at once – you're too small for much variety. Don't wear large patterned fabrics – you'll be swallowed up by the big design.'

On the other hand, **Housewife** magazine of October 1961 told its readers that a taller woman *'can really go to town with bold patterns and interesting textures. She comes into her own with heavy tweeds, basket-weave wools, lacy bouclés, long-haired mohairs, delectable velvets, magnificent brocades – all of which give bulk to the thin woman and help to exaggerate her width. She can wear an explosion of brilliant colours – and striking plaids and checks were made for her.'*

Those *'who have a lot of top'* as the **Boyfriend Annual** of 1961 diplomatically put it, should *'Avoid fussiness on the bodice and never wear too much draping or frills. A little bit of draping is ideal as camouflage, but the moment you start putting on too much you'll end by looking top heavy. Shiny satin will only highlight your bust like a spotlight, and so will the silky jersey types.*

Remember that clinging materials have a habit of clinging. Fine wools and crepes are ideal and so are most of the nylon type fabrics. Suits are good for you, too, provided that they don't have pockets on the bust and that the lapels are long, narrow ones. Wide collars will make you look bigger than you are and so will short sleeves. In fact anything that focuses the eye on the bust is wrong.'

For those *'with heavy hips and a waist that's not all it could be'*, the magazine recommended that *'the straight line is the best; not figure fitting, though, but smooth and easy. Don't have pockets on the hips, don't wear skirts with lots of darts to make you look rounder and never have stripes going round or over-bold patterns. Do choose smooth fabrics, muted colours, gentle*

draping and good jewellery and shoes.'

'If you're skinny you can always comfort yourself that it's fashionable. Hips can never really be too small for fashion, but you can disguise them with a bouffant skirt, which will set off your small waist divinely. Choose dresses with ruched bodices or drapery. Loose fitting dresses with detail at the hemline will also suit you.'

Woman's Weekly in October 1969 stated that *'a good figure depends a great deal on figure control, and that is something which it is up to you to achieve. A controlled figure is one which does not bulge, flop, droop or look ungainly and is pleasing to the eye. Three things play their part in figure control. Diet, exercise and the right foundation.'*

Slimming

Woman's Weekly in October 1969 defined the contemporary diet. *'It means, in modern terms, sensible eating, not half-starving yourself or adopting some eccentric crash programme. It means eating so that you build firm, healthy flesh instead of an excess of fat and keep fit and full of energy.'*

In September 1963 the magazine had advised its readers that *'the number of calories you need depends on your present weight. is a chart showing how many calories you are taking to keep yourself at the weight you are now, presuming you are*

EVERY DAY THIS IS THE NUMBER OF CALORIES A WOMAN NEEDS TO MAINTAIN HER WEIGHT *			
present weight	—at 25 years	—at 45 years	—at 65 years
7 st. 1 lb.	1,900	1,800	1,500
7 st. 12 lb.	2,050	1,950	1,600
8 st. 9 lb.	2,200	2,050	1,750
9 st. 2 lb.	2,300	2,200	1,800
9 st. 6 lb.	2,350	2,200	1,850
10 st. 3 lb.	2,500	2,350	2,000
11 st.	2,600	2,450	2,050
11 st. 11 lb.	2,750	2,600	2,150

CAUTION If your health is in any way below par or you are very much overweight, it is only sensible to ask your doctor's help and advice before beginning any reducing diet.
* Based on moderate activity If your life is very active, add calories; if you lead a sedentary life, subtract calories.

moderately active. If you know you are getting fatter, then you are eating more than the amount of calories you need. Of course, if you want to lose weight you must

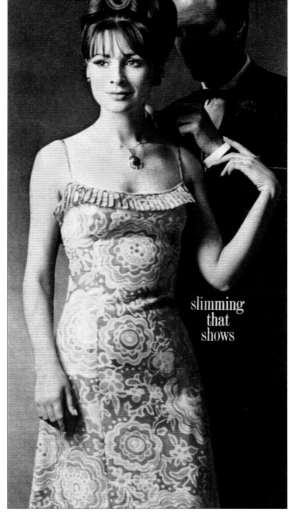

slimming that shows

eat less than you actually need to maintain this weight. Cutting down by 1,000 calories a day should give you a weight loss of about 2 lb. a week. The very lowest diet you should attempt without a doctor's advice is one adding up to 1,000 calories – most women will lose weight steadily on a diet of 1,500.

'Weigh yourself once a week only from now on. If you do not possess your own scales, call into the chemist's at about the same time each week. Slip off your shoes and coat so that your clothes don't count for too much.'

Woman's Realm in March 1963 counselled gradual, sensible eating: '…eat more salad, more fresh fruit and vegetables. In fact, more of every kind of fruit and vegetables, whether frozen, canned, fresh, pre-packed or grown in your own garden.'

Woman's Realm in February 1966 gave a list of basic food for each day: '½ pint of milk; ¾ oz. butter or ½ oz. butter and 1 tablespoon of single cream; three portions of fruit without sugar; or one 1 oz. portion

of low-calorie pudding, 2 oz. bread; 1 egg or 1 oz. cheese; 1 portion of root vegetables; green vegetables or salad; 5 oz. meat or 1 oz. of the meat can be exchanged for 1 egg, 1 oz. of cheese or 2 oz. fish.'

Exercise

One of the first things most authorities insisted upon was improved posture. **Health & Efficiency** magazine in April 1964 advised its readers: 'Look in a full-length mirror. Stand sideways to it, easily and naturally, and note your poise – your posture. Is your head poised well on your shoulders, or does it "poke" forward? And your bust, is it firm and high – or does it sag? Is your back straight – or nearly so? It should be. If none of these natural faults are visible, it is ten to one that you already possess a good figure. If you have any of these faults, something must be done about it.'

'Imagine that you are three inches taller, then, without straining, endeavour to "stand" at this new height. What happens? Your head becomes well poised on the shoulders, which naturally straighten up. The chest is lifted and the bust no longer sags. That little hump in the back and "bulge" in the tummy have disappeared. If you work at a desk, pull the chair up close so that your back can be kept flat against the chair-back. You will not be so tired at the end of the day, and in a week or so, "posture fatigue" will have disappeared. When you are out walking, remember that you are three inches taller than you really are! So walk "tall", if you have to stand for any length of time, stand straight – a natural stance.'

The **Boyfriend Annual** of 1968 also

Left To achieve the perfect, young figure that fashion demanded, most women seemed to be on a permanent diet. July 1966.

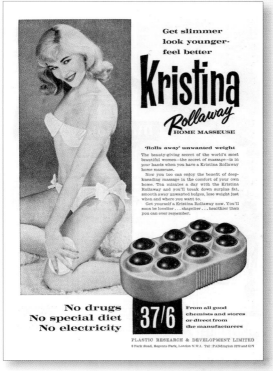

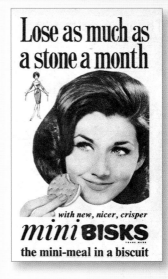

looked at posture: *'If you want to correct a bad habit, try breathing IN to a count of four as deeply as possible, and OUT to a count of eight, as slowly as possible, with whistling lips, to rid your lungs of carbon dioxide. Try this six times, and see how much better you feel. If you practise breathing properly in the garden in warm weather, or by the window at least (open, please!), you'll do yourself twice as much good.'*

Below Exercises, from May 1963.

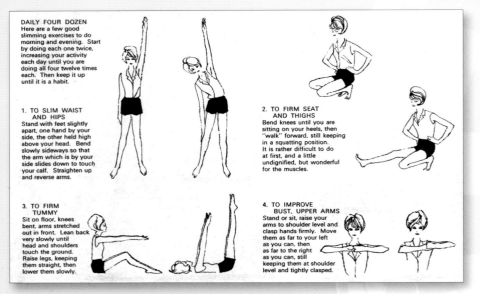

DAILY FOUR DOZEN
Here are a few good slimming exercises to do morning and evening. Start by doing each one twice, increasing your activity each day until you are doing all four twelve times each. Then keep it up until it is a habit.

1. TO SLIM WAIST AND HIPS
Stand with feet slightly apart, one hand by your side, the other held high above your head. Bend slowly sideways so that the arm which is by your side slides down to touch your calf. Straighten up and reverse arms.

2. TO FIRM SEAT AND THIGHS
Bend knees until you are sitting on your heels, then "walk" forward, still keeping in a squatting position. It is rather difficult to do at first, and a little undignified, but wonderful for the muscles.

3. TO FIRM TUMMY
Sit on floor, knees bent, arms stretched out in front. Lean back very slowly until head and shoulders touch the ground. Raise legs, keeping them straight, then lower them slowly.

4. TO IMPROVE BUST, UPPER ARMS
Stand or sit, raise your arms to shoulder level and clasp hands firmly. Move them as far to your left as you can, then as far to the right as you can, still keeping them at shoulder level and tightly clasped.

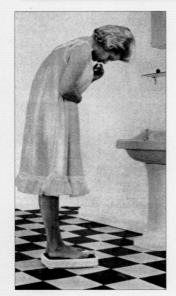

Above In the 1960s losing weight was seen to be about exercise as much as it was diet.

Health & Efficiency suggested an exercise to improve posture: *'Standing erect with the heels together, rise on the toes, then sink rapidly into the full knees bend position. Immediately rise, lowering the arms to the sides as you do so. Repeat 20 times in fairly rapid tempo. It is important that you keep the head up and back straight during this movement, otherwise much of its posture improving value will be lost.'*

Woman magazine in July 1962 advised its readers that: *'Daily walking does wonders for lazy muscles, ensures that contours stay streamlined. Shun the bus and aim for a steady two miles a day.'* **Woman's Weekly** discussed exercise in October 1969: *'…every woman should have a brief repertoire of half-a-dozen exercises or so which will give her a choice of a few to do each day, when she feels like it. The gym-class knees-bend is*

still a super exercise, but remember to rise on your toes first and the back must be held straight with arms at your sides and head erect. So is the one where you raise your elbows, thumbs against the bosom and palms down, and fling your arms simultaneously sideways, each as far as it will go, keeping your arms straight and hands on a level with your shoulders. Terrific for the bust. The rule with any exercise is never to over-do it. Regular, gentle exercising is far more beneficial than violent now-and-again exercises.'*

Woman's Realm took up the theme in December 1968: *'…exercise, every single day, even if it's only for a minute or two. Lie on floor with arms above head, hands flat on floor. Stretch hard, breathing in deeply. Slowly raise arms and legs until toes and fingers meet above your waist, breathing out hard. Lower yourself back to the floor; repeat.'*

Often magazines and books gave more targeted exercises. For thick ankles the **Boyfriend Annual** of 1961 recommended ankle twirling and overhead cycling exercises every day. **Health & Efficiency** recommended this regime for shapely hips and thighs: *'Raise the right arm forwards to a little above shoulder level. Now swing the right leg vigorously upwards, endeavouring to kick the right hand; then immediately swing the leg down and back as far as possible, allowing the knee to bend to give added impetus to the next forward kick. Twenty-five kicks with each leg.'*

Vogue magazine of October 1968 gave the following directions to improve the bust: *'…first stand in front of a mirror so that you can see what you're doing. Turn on some jazz music so that you can do the exercise in syncopated 4/4 time.*

'Start with body in the correct position: stand erect, legs apart; buttocks tucked under; abdomen pulled in; neck and head up, relaxed; shoulders down, relaxed. Bend elbows straight out at the sides and place

hands low on hips, thumbs pressing down at the back, fingers pressing flat on hips in front; you should feel that you're actually holding up and elongating your rib cage, keeping it – and your elbows – as unmovable as possible throughout.

1 Press shoulder straight forward, bring back to centre, press straight back. Bring back to centre. Do 4 times.

2 Same as above, but do not stop at centre, press forward, press back. 4 times.

3 Lift shoulder straight up; press it down, hard. 8 times.

4 Front roll – place shoulder straight forward; roll by lifting it up, bringing it all the way back, then down to centre. Do 4 rolls.

5 Back roll – reverse to no. 4 above. Do 4 rolls.

6 Move shoulder straight forward with sharp accent, let it fall back naturally. 8 times.

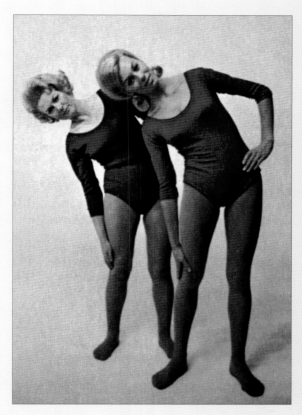

7 Reverse to no. 6, accent back movements only. 8 times.

'Repeat with right shoulder, then both shoulders together.'

And to tone the waist **Woman** in September 1967 recommended: *'Lie flat on floor with arms straight out behind your head. Raise both feet to an angle of twenty degrees and hold for a count of five. From there raise to an angle of forty-five degrees and hold for a count of five. From there raise until they are at a right angle to your body and hold for a count of five. Lower very slowly. Repeat three times. As you get better, raise the count to ten, then twenty…. Still lying on the floor, clasp your hands behind your head then raise straight legs and head and shoulders to make a V shape. Hold this position as long as you can, then relax. Repeat three times.'*

Woman's Weekly in November 1960 even gave exercises for the neck: *'If a double chin is your problem, give this a little firm discipline; using the backs of the hands, slap firmly up under the chin a few times to break down the fatty tissue. Follow this with some head bending and turning exercises, done as slowly as you know how. Drop your head forward on to your chest then raise it again slowly. Now let it fall backwards and raise it slowly upright again. Next, turn it in slow motion from side to side.'*

Foundation Garments

The move towards a slimmer, more youthful outline did not go without protest. As the **Boyfriend Annual** of 1961 put it: *'In spite of*

Running movement for all-over suppling. At position 3 stand still, stretch, then drop quickly into position 4, clapping hands behind back.

Below *What exercise and slimming could not achieve, a good foundation could, 1968.*

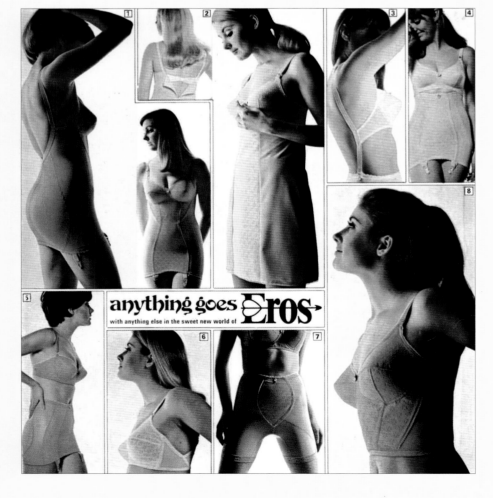

Illustrated: OTHER WONDERFUL TRIUMPH STYLES— IN THE SAME TOP FASHION COLOURS

Czardas Pantie Slimming elastic, with lace and ribbon trim. Small, medium and large. 29/11d.

Miss Triumph Bra In Perlon and lace with firm but gentle undershaping. A, B and C cups. 32–40. £1.
Miss Triumph Girdle In cool, controlling elastic with Perlon front panel. Also in Frosted Jade. 23, 24, 26, 28, at 30/-.

Bra 'n Brief Presenting the trim new swimsuit look, in beautiful lace over Perlon. Bra underwired for perfect support. A and B cups. 32–38. Brief: 24, 26, 28. Also in Frosted Jade and Mistletoe. 2 guineas the set.

Cinch Wisp of a waspie in Perlon with lace trim. Adjustable suspenders. Also in Frosted Jade. 24–30 in inches. £2.

Right *Natural line bra, October 1961.*

Below *By 1966, white was not the only choice in foundations.*

what all the Paris fashion pundits may say, some of us can't and don't want to lose our Venus de Milo figures. Of course, busts can go too far, and the first essential for a big-busted beauty is, of course, a good foundation. If your bust is large, don't be tempted by flimsy, lacy bras. Choose a firmer material with a good wide band underneath to support you. Make sure the bra fits you perfectly before you leave the shop. Whatever the manufacturers may say, I don't believe there is any strapless bra on the market that will support the really large bust. So if you want to keep your figure when you go dancing, you'll just have to choose a dress with covered shoulders. If you want to be daring somewhere buy a dress with a low back – you can buy bras with very good support which will pull down at the back and hook on to your girdle.'

On the other hand, for those who were skinny: *'First, buy yourself a padded bra. You don't need falsies to get a good figure nowadays. So many ordinary bras are padded, and you should always pick one of these instead of the flimsy, skin-tight kind.'*

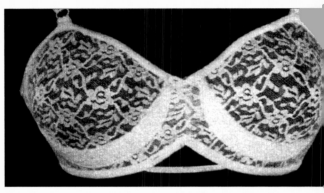

And for those who were short: *'Small girls need to have a smooth line, so if you're small and dumpy it's best to have an all-in-one foundation garment. If you have a slim figure and wear a separate brassière and girdle, make sure the bra gives you a really good uplift.'*

New styles of bra were needed to achieve the softer, line. **Woman's Mirror** in April 1962 reported on them: *'Girls trying the new moulded bras report that they give a beautifully smooth, well-separated line under sweaters. One of the prettiest is made of seamless nylon lace with thin, crescent-shaped under-bust supports. Price: £1 9s 11d.'*

The average age when a girl wore her first bra had now dropped from the mid-teens to about twelve, and bra manufacturers made special models for young wearers. One advert for Berlei bras in June 1960 trumpeted: *'Delightful news for the understanding mother. New bras and girdles specially designed for 11–16 year olds. It is at this age that your daughter's*

anything goes **Eros** →
with anything else in the sweet new world of

young figure begins to need support.' The ad also contained a paragraph that gives an interesting insight into what the girls might be feeling: 'Psychological Note. She wants to wear a bra and girdle anyway – whether she really needs it or not. For it is very important to her to be like the other girls – to belong.'

This expansion of bra-wearing peaked in 1962 with the introduction of the 'sleeping bra', as reported by **Woman's Mirror** in March. *'This garment will be on sale for the first time in Britain this month. The sleeping bra is moulded to the figure, but it's not so constricting as a daytime bra, say the human guinea pigs who've tried it. Already it's selling like wildfire in America. And the manufacturers believe that there are over 13,000,000 women in Britain who'll just love it. That's every bosom-conscious British female between 18 and 60 plus! First in the field of manufacturers are the American firm, Maidenform. Meanwhile, two or three British firms are sitting on the sidelines, waiting to see how the newcomer fares. If sleeping bras are a dizzy success, then expect to see them in every make and price.*

'The sleeping bras you'll be able to buy here are made of nylon tricot and lace in white, black, candy pink and pastel blue. They'll be available in sizes 32-40 in., and will cost around £3. "No, they are not – definitely not – designed only for huge, floppy bosoms," a representative of the makers told me. "They are for anyone with a figure who wants to look after it – and that includes girls of 19 with beautiful bosoms they want to keep that way."

In spite of advances in design, by the mid-1960s dancer turned designer Rudi

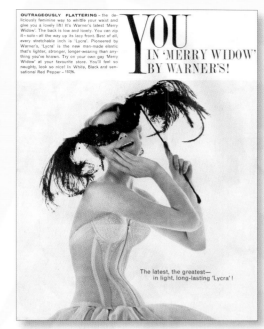

The latest, the greatest— in light, long-lasting 'Lycra'!

Left The 'Merry Widow', April 1965.

Right Q-form bra and girdle by Mary Quant, featuring her trademark daisy.

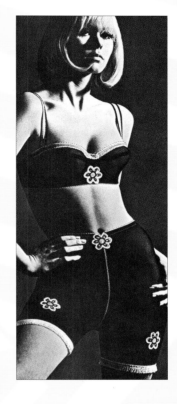

Gernreich could still state that *'Bras have been like something you wear on your head on New Year's Eve.'* Gernreich designed the 'no-bra bra' to underline the body-hugging fashions and the soft clothes of the rest of the decade.

In January 1968 **Woman** magazine described how the *'Frameless crossover "handerchief" bra gives soft round contours – less eye-stopping than reinforced ones'*, and in October 1969 **Woman's Weekly** was recounting that *'Today's demand is for a natural look to the bosom, gently curving but still with a good uplift.'*

Below Black, white, pink, navy, all available, October 1963.

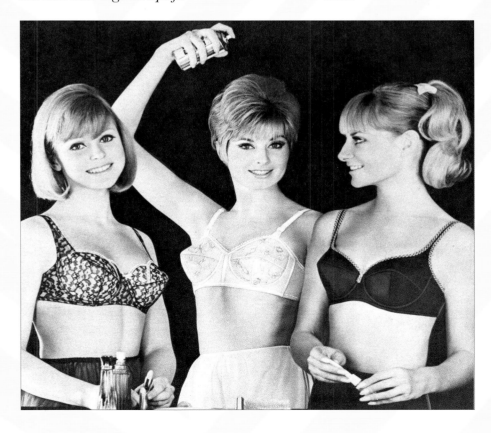

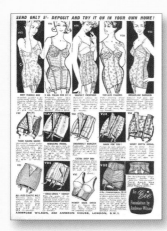

Above April 1965.

Below left *Throughout the sixties, foundations changed from white/flesh colour to a whole range of colours, and from plain to patterned, such as these from April 1969.*

In the early 1960s women virtually all wore a foundation garment of some sort as well as a bra. These included sarong, pull-on and panty-girdles, long-line corselettes and all-in-ones. The long-line was supposed to flatten the stomach and thighs but often produced an unfortunate effect known as the 'mono buttock'.

In 1965 Mary Quant showed her first foundation collection, called Youthlines. This adopted a black-and-white theme, with every brassière related to every girdle.

Foundations and underwear were traditionally offered in black, white or flesh tones, while younger styles might have panels of a small repeated pattern such as dolls or teddy bears. In America, however, coloured foundations in sherry, pink or blue were widely available, as were patterns. However, in Britain there was resistance to the change. **Nova** magazine reported in April 1965 that *'The nicest lingerie colours are still black and white. Coffee and orange are all very well, but they're easily tired of, and anyone will tell you how it complicates your washing. Unless you work at synchronizing it you're stuck with yellow bra, pink slip and brown pants.'*

In spite of such misgivings, colour and pattern began to creep into the ranges of most major manufacturers. At the same time, there were moves afoot that affected the whole range of women's undergarments. **Woman** in January 1968 wrote that *'Permissiveness and the new morality are no friends of the corset manufacturer. They are the social climate in which flourishes the young idea that under your dolly dress it's comfiest to be in the altogether. Tight-laced undies go with a tight-laced society – and no one can say we've been suffering from that.'*

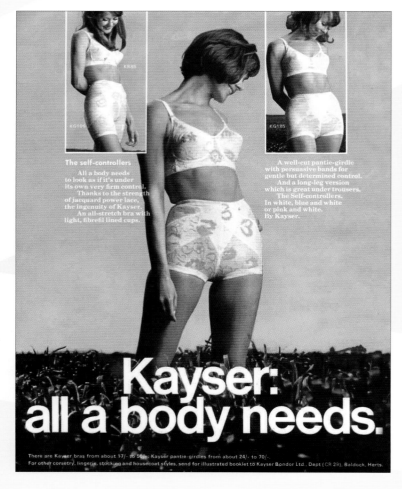

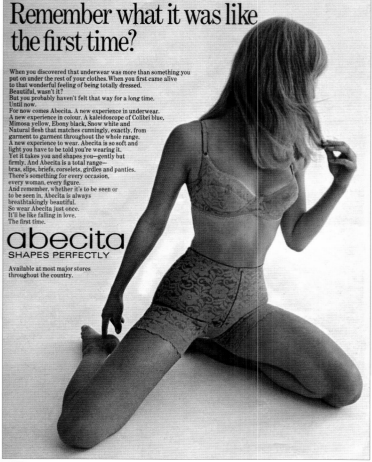

Permissiveness was not the only factor. The growing women's liberation movement associated foundation garments and items such as stockings with women being treated as sex objects. In 1968 there was a famous demonstration at the Miss America contest where bras, girdles, nylons and the like were thrown into a rubbish bin. This gave birth to the idea of burning bras as a sign of protest.

Legs

With legs becoming the focus of the figure, it was important that they looked their best. **Boyfriend Annual** in 1961 stated that: *'Hairy legs are not pretty legs. Fine hair can be rubbed off with a pumice stone, lather your legs well before you start rubbing. A cream depilatory has chemicals that will dissolve the base of the hair. When it is wiped off the hair comes off with it. A wax depilatory is the most effective, but this should be done the first time by an expert in a beauty salon.'*

An alternative approach was described by **Woman** magazine in July 1962: *'Smooth-as-satin legs are a summer "must". Bleaching does the trick for peach-fine fuzz. Paint it with a solution of four tablespoonfuls of 20 volume peroxide, mixed with twelve drops of ammonia to cover legs from thigh tops to ankles. Or make it invisible with a special hair lightener that costs 4s 6d.'*

In May 1967 **Woman** told its readers that *'British girls took to short skirts faster than anyone else, showing the rest of the world just how good it is to look young and swinging. Now everyone wants to be lean and leggy; shorts are getting shorter, legs are looking longer! There's even a new way to walk and stand – a carefree stride look, like a breath of fresh air after our neat mincing steps in stilettos.*

'Mini skirts show off your legs, but they can also show up the imperfections. When you're dark, like Barbara Fry, leg-grooming is as important as a good

hairdo. Barbara shaves her legs every other day to keep them perfectly smooth. She always uses a small hand razor "I've had it for ages. It's one of those plastic ladies' razors, called Nymph. You can get refill blades at the chemist's." She dusts her legs with talc and shaves dry as the growth is so slight after a day or two. Then she pats on some hand cream. Place that's easily missed (but not by onlookers!) is backs of legs. "You have to remember with mini skirts".'

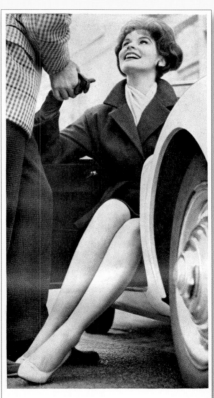

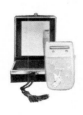

Making what you **have** to do —SOMETHING NICE TO DO!

What a fuss and bother it used to be! Just to achieve a clean, unfuzzy line of leg, and pure white under-arm smoothness. But not any more. The Lady Ronson Superbe is an *electric* shaver, especially for women, which leaves you with skin and pride absolutely intact. No nicks, no scratches, no smarting—just smooth, smooth, beautiful skin. All as quick as a wink. Lady Ronson Superbe will cost you £7.7.0. But you can't measure femininity in terms of money. So save if you have to—but buy it! From leading electrical stores and chemists. 220-240 volts A.C. TV suppressed.

LADY RONSON SUPERBE

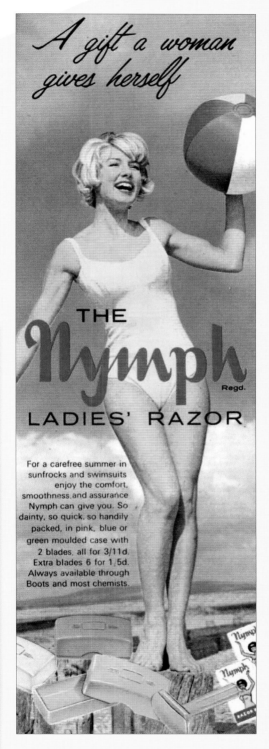

A gift a woman gives herself

THE *Nymph* Regd. LADIES' RAZOR

For a carefree summer in sunfrocks and swimsuits enjoy the comfort, smoothness and assurance Nymph can give you. So dainty, so quick, so handily packed, in pink, blue or green moulded case with 2 blades, all for 3/11d. Extra blades 6 for 1/5d. Always available through Boots and most chemists.

Above *Traditional Nymph ladies' razor, June 1961.*

Left *Short hemlines needed smooth legs: ladies' electric shaver, July 1966.*

MAKE UP AND COSMETICS

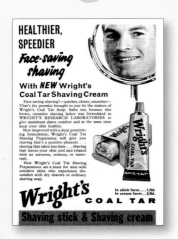

HEALTHIER, SPEEDIER *Face-saving shaving* With *NEW* Wright's Coal Tar Shaving Cream

Face-saving shaving!—quicker, closer, smoother—That's the promise brought to you by the makers of Wright's Coal Tar Soap. Safer too, because this better, creamier shaving lather was formulated in WRIGHT'S RESEARCH LABORATORIES to give maximum shave comfort and at the same time keep your skin healthy.

Now improved with a deep penetrating formulation, Wright's Coal Tar Shaving Preparation will give you shaving that's a positive pleasure . . . shaving that takes less time . . . shaving that leaves your skin cool and relaxed with no soreness, redness, or razor-rash.

New Wright's Coal Tar Shaving Preparations are a must for men with sensitive skins who experience discomfort with dry shavers or ordinary shaving soap.

In stick form . . . 1/5d. In cream form . . 2/8d.

Wright's COAL TAR

Shaving stick & Shaving cream

Above At the start of the decade, the range of men's toiletries was very limited, January 1962.

Right Aftershave, November 1962, at this time, definitely only for the younger generation.

Top right, above December 1967, and Chanel are even producing a cologne for men – it was the end of an era where 'real men' smelt of carbolic soap or sweat.

Men

At the start of the 1960s men's toiletries were limited in range, consisting almost entirely of hair cream and shaving soap, shaving cream and aerosol shaving soap. Aftershave lotion was getting popular with younger men – the most sought-after brands included Old Spice and later Brut – while the increasing use of electric razors provided a market for pre-electric shave lotion.

Once the concept of men smelling of anything other than sweat or carbolic soap was established, other forms of toiletries specifically formulated for men, such as deodorant, cologne and talc, began to be accepted. In December 1966, for instance, Mennen advertised body talc, aftershave, aerosol shave cream, stick deodorant and electric pre-shave lotion. Many of these were not bought by the men themselves, but were given to them as birthday or Christmas presents.

The better brands took off, and not just for men. **Boyfriend** magazine in 1965 noted that *'It seems more and more girls will start pinching their boyfriends' after-shave lotions. Lots of them do already, of course, and it's not surprising. Men have been smelling better and better for some time now.'*

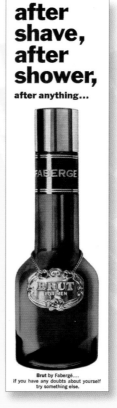

after shave, after shower, after anything...

FABERGE

BRUT FOR MEN

Brut by Fabergé... if you have any doubts about yourself try something else.

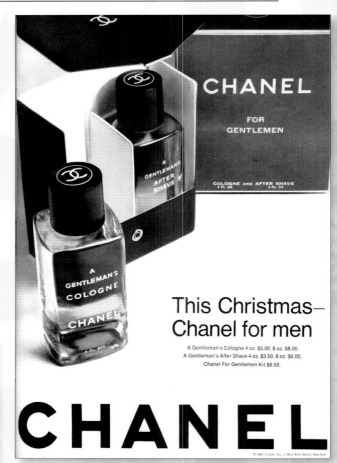

CHANEL FOR GENTLEMEN
COLOGNE AND AFTER SHAVE

A GENTLEMAN'S AFTER SHAVE

A GENTLEMAN'S COLOGNE

CHANEL

This Christmas— Chanel for men

A Gentleman's Cologne 4 oz. $5.00. 8 oz. $8.00.
A Gentleman's After Shave 4 oz. $3.50. 8 oz. $6.00.
Chanel For Gentlemen Kit $8.50.

CHANEL

Women

1960 Applying make-up was an art. **House Wife** magazine advised its readers that *'If using a moisture base, apply it slowly and evenly. Spot the powder foundation in small drops on the forehead, nose, cheekbones and chin, then blend carefully so that you get a fine, even film. Apply powder by pressing it on generously with a firm rolling movement.'*

Lipstick was mainly red or peach in colour; Helena Rubinstein's range included, 'Heart of Peach, Heart of Cherry, Heart of

Coral, Heart of Red, Heart of Pink and Heart of Rose Red'.

Eye make-up was still considered by some to be a little 'racy'. However, the fashion was for a younger look, and the focus of the face moved from the lips to the eyes, which had to look as large and round as possible. February's **Woman magazine** advised that *'If you're wary of eye make-up, but secretly long to try it, a complete eye make-up pack has just been brought out for only 2s 3d. It consists of two eye-shadow shades and two mascara shades with a brush in a tiny box, and comes in three colour ranges – for brown, blue or grey eyes. There's an exciting new idea in eye pencils, too – outsize ones in pastel colours that are easier to use than eyeshadow, stay on better because they're not greasy. Price is 3s 8d.'*

The magazine also advised: *'Some firms make lipstick refills that look good enough to use on their own – 6s 6d buys you a prettily cased refill. And once you've found a shade you want to go on using, you can graduate to a proper case. It takes a lot of time and testing to find the scent that's just "you": so it's*

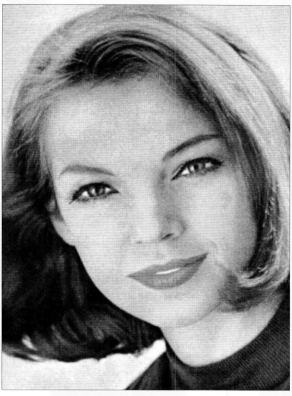

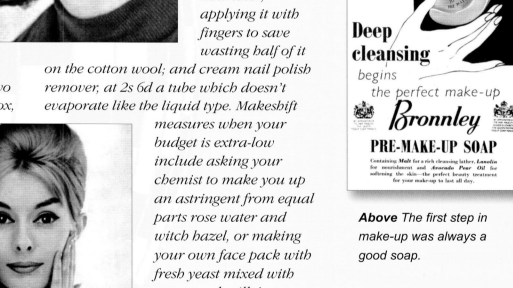

cheaper to buy miniature bottles. Several top French perfume houses sell exciting fragrances in tiny bottles – two of the best ranges cost only 5s 6d and 7s. Just like love, when the right scent hits you, you'll know it.'

Woman also gave substitutes: *'…you can use a baby lotion priced 1s 8½d as a cleanser and a nourisher, applying it with fingers to save wasting half of it on the cotton wool; and cream nail polish remover, at 2s 6d a tube which doesn't evaporate like the liquid type. Makeshift measures when your budget is extra-low include asking your chemist to make you up an astringent from equal parts rose water and witch hazel, or making your own face pack with fresh yeast mixed with water and milk.'*

1961 Woman's Weekly told its readers that *'Make-up is not just a set of creams and powders which suit your skin texture and colouring – it is a look, a fashion which changes each year and each season just as our clothes change. If you want to be one of the* smart set, you must keep up with what is new in make-up. Not all the latest ideas or the newest shades will suit you, of course.'

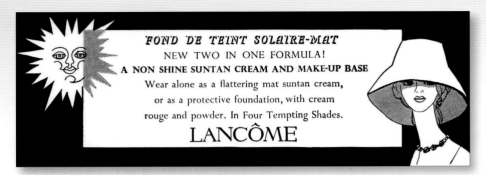

FOND DE TEINT SOLAIRE-MAT
NEW TWO IN ONE FORMULA!
A NON SHINE SUNTAN CREAM AND MAKE-UP BASE
Wear alone as a flattering mat suntan cream,
or as a protective foundation, with cream
rouge and powder. In Four Tempting Shades.
LANCÔME

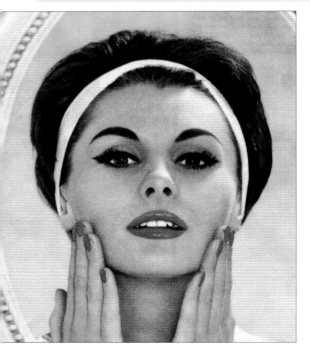

Above Heavy mascara and eye shadow, and the lips and nails are unashamedly bright red, April 1961.

Right Advert from June 1961. Notice the subdued lipstick on the left is for 'young, tender days'. As the fashionable look became a youthful one, so such muted lipstick colours became all the rage.

The magazine looked at make-up for the summer: *'If you do not tan, you can wear a tinted foundation – and very flattering they are, too. Smartest this Summer is a beige-tinted one, subtle, neutral, close to the natural tones of the skin. For a natural, open-air look, don't powder over a tinted foundation – leave the skin looking smooth and polished. You can add a hint more brown with a foundation just that much deeper, but don't risk one so deep you look like a streaked orange! If you are hoping to tan, wear only a transparent moisturising cream or a sun-filter cream.'*

On powder: *'…find a muted tone to match foundation and keep it mostly for after-dark or more formal wear. Powder-cake used over a foundation looks slightly smoother and less made-up in strong sunshine.… Rouge has made a comeback this season.… Eyes may still be top news, but I have always felt that a pale, dead-pan skin is unflattering. Rouge, of course, mustn't show. Only you know you are wearing it – others just remark how marvellously well you are looking! You'll*

find liquid rouge particularly subtle. Liquid (or cream) rouge goes on over foundation, before any powder. Buy it to tone with your lipstick shade so that it gives your skin an apricot, coral or pinky glow, which blends with your make-up.'

Woman's Journal advised its readers that the *'Newest look for eyes is a fine line drawn along the upper lids immediately above lashes or in a beguiling, tilting triangle at the eye corner.'* It added that *'Paris has gone all misty-eyed in Winter for party make-up. Lashes are soft, sooty black against deeply shadowed eyelids, lightened with a faint gleam of pearl.'*

Woman's Weekly declared that *'Eye make-up is still all-important to a fashionable appearance, so please don't neglect to use it. In fact, when in a hurry, it is almost better to let skin make-up go and draw a pair of dazzling eyes.*

'Eye shadow as a cream is being superseded by liquid eye-liners which are painted on with a small brush. Learn to do this and you can enhance your eyes

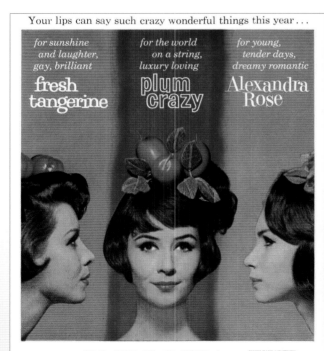

Your lips can say such crazy wonderful things this year…

for sunshine and laughter, gay, brilliant
fresh tangerine

for the world on a string, luxury loving
plum crazy

for young, tender days, dreamy romantic
Alexandra Rose

INNOXA
YOUR WORLD OF BEAUTY IN A WORD

JEWELFAST LIPSTICKS
Lustrous, indelible.
Lipstick complete 5/-
In gold and silver case 7/6

wonderfully. Most fashionable shades are turquoise and mauve. You paint the eye shadow along the upper lashes and extend it into little upward turning wings. Differently shaped eyes can take different shadow shapes – have fun making fatter or thinner, longer or shorter wings to see which is most effective.

'If you still prefer eye shadow which is fingered on, there is a pretty palette with a range of summer blues and greens. Perhaps even simpler to apply are stick shadows – again, sky blues and sea greens are pretty choices for a sunny day. Sophisticates can make up after-dark eyes with muted browns and beiges.

'For your eyelashes you need mascara. Don't forget that even the darkest lashes have paler tips and so will look longer when made up.

'For the eyebrows, have an eye-brow pencil. Newest are the soft, crayon types which draw on natural looking lines. These velvety-soft "leads" are also fine for drawing dark lines close along the eyelashes when you want your eyes to look their largest and most brilliant.'

Eye make-up colours that year included 'twin shadow stick' by Miners in lilac/turquoise, Revlon frosted shadow in gold bronze, Gala shadow stick in pearl shades: olive, gold, beige, and brown, Helena Rubinstein's liquid eye liner in black, brown, blue, green, or violet, and Coty liquid eyeliner in 'Exciting Green' and 'Shimmering Blue'.

Lips became paler to focus attention on the eyes. **Woman's Weekly** in June gave its readers advice on the latest shades of lipstick: 'Shades are all pale, not competing too much with the warm tints of the skin and the big, big eyes. Choose from a whole gamut of new shades – roses of many tints, peaches, nectarines, corals, oranges and one or two spicy reds. There are also plenty of muted beigey tones for those who like the very latest – and have the courage to wear it.

'On the whole, wear the warmer, golden pinks and reds if your skin tends to tan; the cool, blue-pinks if you expect to stay pale. But blondes can wear the softer nectarine shades and brunettes do look wonderful in pink.'

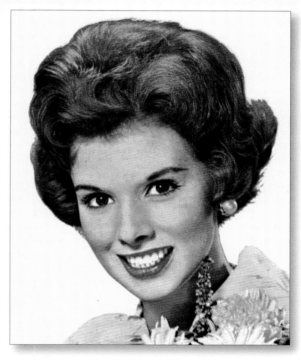

Left April 1962, a more natural look, but still an emphasis on the lips.

1962 **Men Only** magazine reported on make-up wearing; it found that teenagers spent the most on make-up – an average of £8 a year each – and that 'The general rule is against much rouge – only seven women in a hundred habitually wear it now. Since pallor is fashionable, a general appearance of ghostliness cannot be judged intentionally weird, though the clinching feature is eye make-up. Eyes are normally more heavily made up today – five women use eye shadow now for every one five years ago. A female who fiercely blocks in the bottom of her eyes as well as the lashes is "normal" if she is 15 (when everyone does it) and subnormal if she is over 21. As soon as women get married they ease off make-up, eventually dropping to about a third of their old consumption.'

Woman's Journal that summer gave descriptions of the eye cosmetics available,

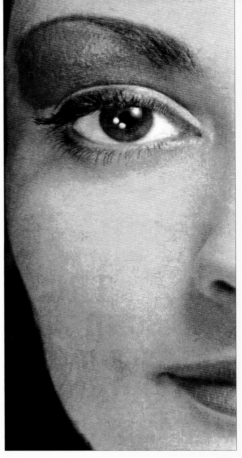
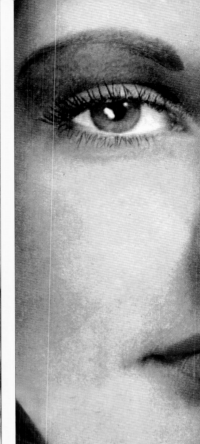

Right The new heavily-accentuated eye make up January 1962.

and how they should be used: 'The beatnik eye – heavily smouldering, dark darling of the past year – strikes the same dated note today as the eye devoid of any artifice. What, then, is the new technique? Pale, wonderful colours which emphasise, but do not darken, a deft hand with an eye-liner and a light but steady touch with the mascara – worth using as carefully as though it costs guineas a go. The effect – light and ephemeral, natural and extremely pretty!

'Eye-shadows come in several forms. There are cream shadows, which are patted on with the finger-tips, blending lightly all over the lids and away to nothing at the brow-line; and shadow sticks, firmer than cream shadow and making a more definite line – usually in shimmering, brighter shades which are stroked on the outer corners of the eyes to emphasise the eye colour. Newest of all, are the shadows in fluid cream or cream powder form which colour the lids with a beautifully matt finish.

'Eye-liners give definition to the eye, play up the colour and shape. Liners can be in pencil or in liquid form – the

Below 'Young' lipstick colours, August 1962.

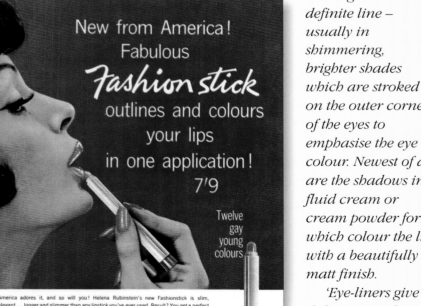

New from America! Fabulous *Fashion stick* outlines and colours your lips in one application! 7'9

Twelve gay young colours

America adores it, and so will you! Helena Rubinstein's new Fashionstick is slim, elegant... longer and slimmer than any lipstick you've ever used. Result? You get a perfect outline and the loveliest colour on your lips in one application. Perfect! So is the texture. Soft and smooth with a deep, rich sheen that makes the colour glow! 12 of fashion's gayest young colours to choose from, too. At your favourite beauty counter *now*. Fashionstick Standard Case 7/9. Golden de Luxe Case 12/6. Refills to fit either case 5/6.

Helena Rubinstein

latter to be painted on with a thin sable brush, applied while stretching the eyelid taut with the other hand. Always draw the line close to the roots of the lashes and don't be afraid to experiment with the shape of the line – a little illusory editing can do wonderful things for minor imperfections of shape. For instance, a tapered crescent across the upper lash-line makes small eyes rounder, larger; a line that thickens towards the outer edge makes eyes seem almond-shaped. Too-close eyes should be outlined only from the centre out.

'Eyebrow pencils – however beautifully you make up your eyes, they will appear imperfectly groomed unless your brows are kept tidy in a smooth, precisely etched outline. To tidy up stray hairs, tweak from underneath the brow-line – never alter the top curve of the brow. Nine eyes out of ten are improved by brows that are a little longer, so practise, practise, practise until you can feather-stitch a realistically perfect shape with little eye-fooling strokes. As for colours, use two shades to keep the effect soft and subtle – brown and black if you are dark, brown and grey if you are in-between, grey and light chestnut if you are fair or reddish.

'Mascaras – the final detail, several thin coats of mascara – far more effective than one thick layer. Brush once all over all the lashes, upper and lower lid, and then add three extra applications on the top lashes, brushing outwards and upwards at the outer corners. Traditional block mascara applied with a dampened brush is quick and easy to use – cream mascara gives a thick, silky appearance to sparse lashes and helps to make them supple and glossy. For touching-up purposes – the new spiral mascaras, which separate, colour and curl the lashes!'

The magazine gave instructions on how to achieve for the latest look in eye make up: '1 Brows – pluck stray hairs from under brows, or have an expert improve the whole brow-line to one you can copy and keep. Pencil goes on in light strokes: then comb brows for that really groomed look.

2 Eye-defining lines need plenty of practice. Take pencil or liquid line from not-quite inner corner to just beyond outer corner of eye, above lashes. Finish line subtly, by tilting it slightly upwards. If you pencil, brush over the line to soften it. With liquid liner, don't let line end in a blob!

3 False lashes make yours seem twice as thick. Trim fakes so they don't look outrageously long; cut the strip of lashes to less than eye-length, then smear with fixative. Hold strip with tweezers – and place on lid, on top of your own lashes. Tweezer in position before glue gets firm.

4 Shadow is worked in with finger or sable brush: use most colour close to lashes, less as it goes brow-wards. (Eyes small? Leave lid colour free, or stroke on white lipstick. Concentrate colour shadow from upper lid to eyebrow.) Finally, pat lightly with powdered cotton wool to set shadow.

5 Mascara goes on top of upper lashes first, then underneath, with brush or applicator curling lashes up and outwards.

Paint on two coats, then separate lashes with a dry brush. On lower lashes go gently please – just a thin coat at outer corners. Remember! Use block mascara nearly dry.

6 Colour-picking is fun – brown eyes are great with greens, browns, "muddy" shadows. Match blue iris with blue, or go green, mauve, turquoise. Grey-blue eyes need soft green, not cold blue. High-colour complexions avoid mauves – try turquoise, light green, or cool grey.'

'Why stick with just one colour when two can give your regular make-up a quick change of mood – as above! We painted on two black lines – one close to lashes, one high on the lid. Between them goes white shadow; 'twixt upper line and eyebrow – take crazy brown shadow. Try this two-toning tactic with blue, white, green, white – or light – and dark shades of one colour.'

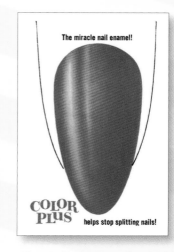

Above 'Color Plus' for nails, by Lanolin Plus.

1963

In January **Modern Woman** made predictions for 1963: 'In will come the clear Impressionist colours for lips and eyes. Out go the orange and apricot toned lipsticks. In their place we'll see an exciting array of brighter, clearer pinks. Clear pink nail polish will be the theme for fingertips, too. 'Out go the blue and green eyeshadows. In – iris, beige, brown and grey with matching shades of eyeliner. Eyes will still be dominant – but with slightly less eyeliner than we've been wearing. The pale translucent complexion make-up will stay, too, with one addition; we'll take to wearing that long neglected cosmetic – rouge. (Now's the time to start learning how to blend it below cheekbones to add interesting hollows to a too-round face,

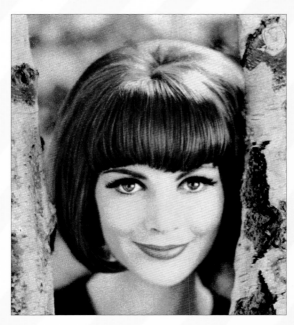

Above The 'look' of 1963.

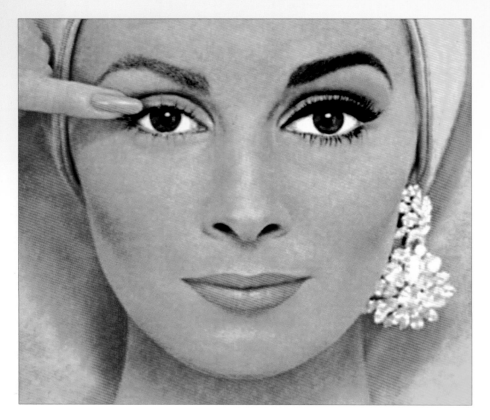

Above October 1963, and the eyes are definitely taking over as the centre of attention.

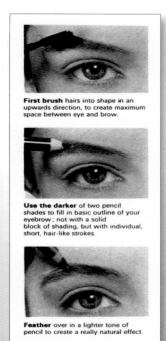

First brush hairs into shape in an upwards direction, to create maximum space between eye and brow.

Use the darker of two pencil shades to fill in basic outline of your eyebrow; not with a solid block of shading, but with individual, short, hair-like strokes.

Feather over in a lighter tone of pencil to create a really natural effect.

Above Applying eyebrow make up, October 1963.

over cheekbones to dramatise contours and along the jawline to soften a long, lean face.) I expect to see an increased use of false eyelashes.'

In October **Woman magazine** looked at eyebrows, stating that *'One minute a day to pencil them and one session a week shaping them gives you pretty brows. The fashion look, most attractive for brows, is the natural look: gentle arcs no more than a shade or two darker than the hair colouring.*

'If brows are naturally well shaped, pluck only to tidy away a few stragglers under the brow or over the nose. Never over-pluck the eyebrows. Dark-haired girls often need no pencil – just a spot of Vaseline, applied with a brush, keeps brows neat. Where hairs are too sparse or very fair, brows can be emphasized with short, hair-like pencil strokes.

'Crayon pencils cost from 1s 6d upwards. They must be kept well sharpened for an efficient job. More expensive – but time-saving and efficient – are the very fine line

pencils which have a self-sharpener. Mascara can be used instead of pencil or liquid when brows are naturally well shaped and hairs are not sparse. Brush it on to the hairs only for the most natural effect.'

Flair magazine that October suggested colours for a girl with dark auburn hair, green eyes and pale skin: turquoise or green eye shadow, green mascara and a brownish-red lipstick by day, and a golden pink lipstick at night.

1964 The **Boyfriend Annual** that summer looked at day and evening make-up for a busy working girl: *'Morning – Rub some colourless moisturiser into your face, or some invisible cream foundation. Powder generously and rub off the excess with a dab of cotton wool.*

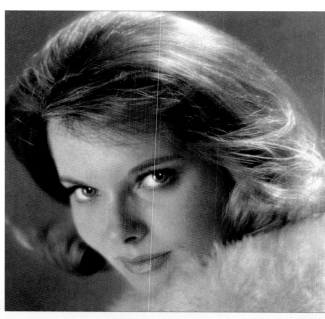

'Now for your evening make-up. Put on some green foundation cream, and cover with beige powder. For a shiny evening look, apply some moisturiser, then put on a foundation that does not need powder. Don't use rouge with this make-up. Rouge looks harsh unless it is powdered over.'

Again, the eyes were most important: *'If, in spite of a reasonably early bed and good* ventilation, you still frequently wake up with bags under your eyes, give yourself a witch-hazel treatment for five minutes before you pop out of bed. Soak a wad of cotton wool in witch-hazel and lay it over your shut eyes. It will take away your sleepy heaviness and tighten up the muscles round your eyes. You should, while you were eating your breakfast, have dabbed the skin under your eyes with milk. During break-fast it would have dried, and by the time you come to wash your face prior to making up, the milk will have tightened the skin.'

'Don't use liquid eye-liner first thing in the morning unless you are extremely skilful with it. It needs a good twenty minutes to put it on properly and to let it dry. Use an ordinary eye pencil for a faint line around your lids, and for a flick up at the corners. Mascara is not the best thing for a day at work – it often runs. And eye-shadow should be kept to a minimum – perhaps a touch of pale blue or pale green. But nothing brighter, and certainly not a shiny shadow.

'False lashes are difficult to put on well. If you wear them, make sure you have tried them on and trimmed them to suit your face, before you go out in them. Easier to put on is black lash fluff, which comes from Switzerland. It is fairly expensive still, but no doubt the price will go down later. Mascara your lashes with a roller first. Then stroke the fluff on to your lashes, and leave it for two minutes to set. Then roller them into place with some more mascara.

'For a very special evening look, use two tones of eye-shadow. Try a deep tone of blue or green or turquoise on the lids, then fade in grey or brown up to the eyebrows. Paint a long line of eye-liner on your upper lids, and a short line from centre to outer end of the lower lids. Flick gently upwards from the upper lids.'

And for the mouth: 'Take a paint brush and outline your mouth with a darker shade of lipstick than you use for the rest of

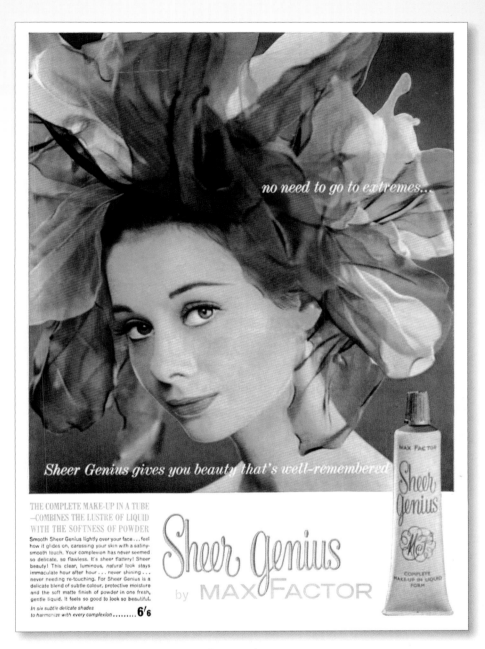

no need to go to extremes...

Sheer Genius gives you beauty that's well-remembered

THE COMPLETE MAKE-UP IN A TUBE —COMBINES THE LUSTRE OF LIQUID WITH THE SOFTNESS OF POWDER

Smooth Sheer Genius lightly over your face...feel how it glides on, caressing your skin with a satiny-smooth touch. Your complexion has never seemed so delicate, so flawless. It's sheer flattery! Sheer beauty! This clear, luminous, natural look stays immaculate hour after hour...never shining... never needing re-touching. For Sheer Genius is a delicate blend of subtle colour, protective moisture and the soft matte finish of powder in one fresh, gentle liquid. It feels so good to look so beautiful. In six subtle delicate shades to harmonize with every complexion........**6/6**

Sheer Genius by MAX FACTOR

MAX FACTOR
Sheer Genius
COMPLETE MAKE-UP IN LIQUID FORM

your mouth. Fill in the gap with a pink or light coral shade. NEVER paint the whole of your mouth in a dark red for daytime.'

Woman's Journal took up the subject of lipstick: 'A new look at lipstick sees the pale, "barely" colours still up at the winning post, but with clear, medium reds coming in a close second and possible favourites for the autumn colour stakes. The youngest way to wear red comes from Le Rouge Baiser in their pearlised lipstick formula – a clever colour combination of plain and pearl that lets lips glisten through a gentle warmth of

Above Softer lips, bigger eyes, September 1964.

colour. There are several soft reds in the pearlised range including the new "Peach Cream". Germaine Monteil's red forecast is "Prelude" and "Ambiance". For young lips that still prefer the off-beat pinks and browns, there's sugar-pink "Lollipops and Roses" from Innoxa, together with "Wild Chinchilla", verging on caramel.'

Below Lipstick colours, December 1964.

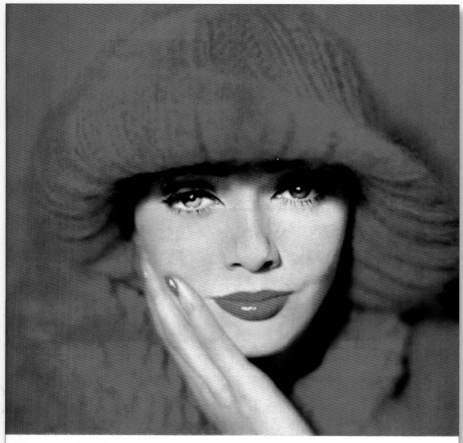

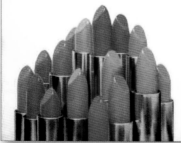

Tender, colourful, smooth, brilliant, creamy, m-mmmm lipstick by Revlon.

It glides on fashionably, deliciously, temptingly. Doesn't streak, smear, cake or fade. Long-lasting flattery! Have you tried it lately?

Lipstick by Revlon in "Colors Unlimited."
She's wearing fashion's latest shade: 'Revlon's Stormy Pink'

Modern Woman that October gave advice on make up to go with the autumn fashions: 'Make-up and hairstyles have undergone subtle changes to complete the 'old fashioned' look for the coming season.

This season's demure old-fashioned look calls for a new beauty. Complexions have all the romantic beauty of a cameo portrait – porcelain clear skin, pink cheeks, large shining eyes.

'Choose your foundation and powder carefully, avoiding the tans, or honeys, or even the peach tones unless the very light ones particularly suit your individual colouring. Wear instead cream shades, or best of all, pinky colours to complement the exciting new range of lipstick colours. Blue reds are back, but not in the harsh, improbable shades we used to wear. They come in a wonderful range to tone with all the latest fashion colours. Remember that your foundation should always be darker by one shade than your powder. This gives a smooth, flatteringly translucent look. Pick your foundation slightly darker than the final colour you want, and your powder in a shade slightly lighter.

'Eyelashes are in the limelight just now – and the new filament mascaras will give them extra thickness and length.

'Of the new fashion colours purple is one of the most dramatic and exciting, wonderful on redheads, and it gives all of us a chance to go on using a pink lipstick if we happen to prefer it. But not the baby pink you wore in the summer; be sure it is one of the new lively pinks laced with a kind of blue – try Lancaster Montana, Coty's French Spice, Leichner Cyclamen Rose.

'It is better not to match dark Plum, as this is a sombre colour for lipstick, but a lighter lipstick with a matching amount of blue in it will blend in, and you might take a look at Innoxa Plum Crazy, Helena Rubinstein's Tender Pink and Estée Lauder's Swiss Strawberry.

'Bottle green gives more scope for choice. Lighter blue reds will blend in well, like Goya Chinese Pink or Revlon Butterfly Pink. Or those who like to vary the season's blue-red rule could use a clear but strong red.

'With mustard, blue-reds vanish. Here the orange, gold and coral shades take over, in darker versions than we have seen for a long time.

'Of all the colours we will be wearing this autumn, crimson is probably the easiest and most wearable for all of us, whether blonde, brunette or redhead. Whenever possible, match it exactly with your lipstick.'

1965 Woman magazine gave advice for skin care: 'Oil, salt and lemon – that's my recipe for a soft skin. About once a fortnight I cover my face with baby oil, then rub over with salt and lemon juice mixed into a paste.' While to lighten the skin, the magazine recommended that you 'mix the juice with egg to cleanse and tone your face. Method: mix a little lemon juice with the yolk of an egg. Leave on for a few minutes. Remove with egg white, beaten to a froth. Splash face with cold water.'

Once again, eyes were the subject of much advice; **Woman** gave its readers these tips: 'For larger-looking eyes try this: white eyeshadow on upper lids, shadow to match

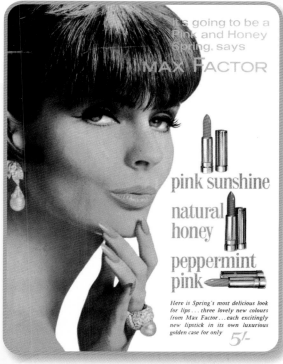

Left Lighter shades for both lipstick and nails, 1965.

your eyes on top, brown shading above in the crease of the eye, make lashes look really thick by putting on mascara then powdering them, and adding a couple more coats of mascara. Use a toothbrush for putting on mascara – it goes on better that way. Short false lashes look more natural than mascara – But they're hard on your own lashes – so brush regularly with olive oil. Final touch for a big night out: perfume brushed on eyebrows – it gives them a gleam, takes off that powdery look.'

Brides magazine that autumn gave advice for eye make-up on the big day: 'Turquoise eyeshadow was applied to the outer half of the lid and powdered with talc (a useful tip, because it sets without discolouring the shade), then more turquoise was brushed on. The lids were lined behind the lashes with "French Green". Black Cotymatic Mascara made lashes lusciously long. Brows were rubbed lightly with grey eyebrow pencil.'

Woman also gave advice on lipstick. 'I treat my lips while I sleep: rub in Vaseline at bedtime – my lipstick goes on better that way.'

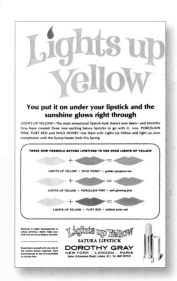

Above Lipstick from April 1965.

Left Heavy owl eyes, April 1965.

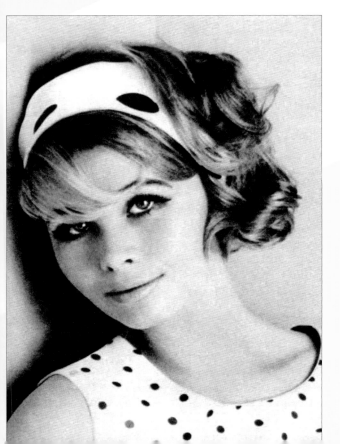

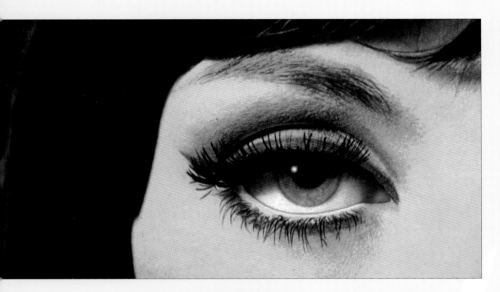

Above Eye make up, October 1966.

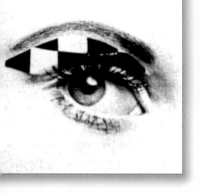

Above The op art look for eyes January 1966.

Right By 1967 the fashion for jazzy colours and op art designs was giving way to a softer, more romantic look.

1966 The Op Art fashion stretched to eye-shadow. At Elizabeth Arden customers could have squares drawn on their eyelids and filled in with colour. **Vanity Fair** suggested a quick, cheap alternative: '… *make your op-art eyelids instantly. We did these with racing sticky tape – 1966 things have to be quick. Reinforce the stickiness with eyelash glue.*'

The nails were perfect for the Op Art look, and **Vanity Fair** also gave suggestions for them: '*Miner's Pop-art version: black or white polish with white or black transfers fixed with colourless base. Notice too Cyclax Pearl Sheen or the exciting back-to-the-thirties Chitibean by Revlon, a vivid plum. The demise of pale tones means better-groomed nails, with colour more carefully applied – dark colours show every brush waver at the cuticle. This could mean the return of the half-moon in 1966.*'

1966 even saw the comeback of an eighteenth-century fashion – the beauty spot. **Vanity Fair** suggested: '…*make a stick-on mole from brown felt. Round, shaped like a tiny heart, or, for parties, a sequin-centred flower. Very flattering. Stick them with eyelash fixative near an eye or below the mouth.*' Or if this was too daring, you might '*add sparkle to your shell-like ears with a framing row of silver sequins. Parties only though, please, and stick them with eyelash glue and tweezers. They catch the light and throw off the most 1966 sparks. Try mother-of pearl sequins too.*'

In April Mary Quant launched a new range of cosmetics. '*All the eye shadows are subtle "sludgy" colours that make eyes look huge. Bright, primitive colours for eyes and mouth are out, so far as my cosmetic collection is concerned.*'

1967 In September **Woman** magazine investigated the latest trends in make-up. '*The accent is on eyes: they're soft, dewy and very expressive. It's still the tawny story for skin, but maybe a tone or two peachier. The newest trend in powders: translucent see-throughs that turn shine to peach-skin; don't build up colour or texture. Shading (to shape as well as to add life and colour to skin) is still top news, but our experts all agreed that it should be blended to look like a bloom on the skin – never a blotch. The logical choice: warm peachy beige.*

'*20 plus eye make-up should be softly misted. Eyeshadow runs the gamut from violet to golden olive. Blues and greens are most popular. Eyeliners and mascaras are mainly teamed to eyeshadow, adding richer flirtier emphasis to natural eye colour. Lips follow suit with skin – tawny tones with a hint of pink.*'

The magazine gave its readers directions for achieving a new, elegant look: '…*with*

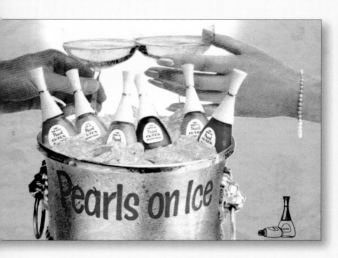

Pearls on Ice

your basic eye shade, sparkling with silver, darkening with grey, toning in liner and lashes.'

Another edition of **Woman** featured the 'switched-on look' for younger, more fashionable women. 'Basically beige, it has glowing warm-skinned appeal with white, silver or gold highlighters emphasizing cheek-bones, forehead or chin. Basically, too, it's a no-powder look, although frosted powders or translucents over-topping cream foundation can be used to get the same sheeny switched-on effect. Emphasis is on a "total" look with eye and lip colour muted to complement subtle green and russet fashion shades of autumn. For eyes: soft greys, blues and browns for shadow, liner and mascara. Frosted or matt shadows will blend into silver, gold, or white sheeners from eyelid crease to brow. Fake lashes? Sometimes … but the choice is for lighter and more natural-looking fakes. For lips: a hint of beigey pink, with built-in or added sheen.'

While some clothes designers had plumped for the longer hemlines, Courrèges, Rabanne and Ungaro stayed loyal to the extremely short mini. This was known as the 'bare as you dare' style, which prompted Coty to introduce a new line of cosmetics – body paint.

warm, peach-tone colouring, pastel-shaded eyes, vibrant clear lips.
1. Smooth foundation upwards from base of neck; all over face; blend carefully at jaw-line.
2. Lightener is finger-painted beneath eyes to cover any tiny lines or shadow.
3. Brush rouge along cheekbones, blend with foundation and powder.
4. Fluff powder all over face and neck in upward pats with cotton wool. Smooth off surplus with brush or tissue in downward movement.
5. Brush dark-tone shading beneath chin in half-moon shape.

'Discussing lip colours, the pale pinks to the poppy reds suit every age. Any blotting must not be seen to have been done.'

In May, **Woman** gave ideas for eye-shadow. 'Start with milky blue basic shade, slicked over lids, topped with a breath of silver, deepened with grey in a curve above lid, silvered again winging up to brows. (Top lashes aflutter with blue above, smokey grey or jet below. Liner a deep, rich blue.) Or take a soft sea green, gentle lilac or toasty brown as

Far left Wet look lipstick was matched with pearly nail varnish.

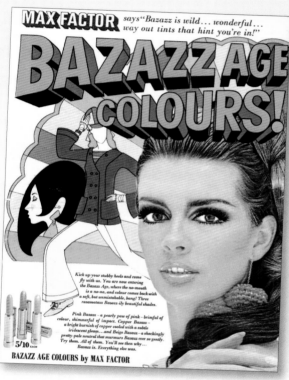

MAX FACTOR says "Bazazz is wild… wonderful … way out tints that hint you're in!"

BAZAZZ AGE COLOURS!

Kick up your stubby heels and come fly with us. You are now entering the Bazazz Age, where the na-mouth is a na-no, and colour comes back with a soft, but unmistakable, bang! Three razamazazz Bazazz-ily beautiful shades.

Pink Bazazz – a pearly paw of pink – brimful of colour, shimmerful of impact. Copper Bazazz – a bright burnish of copper cooled with a subtle iridescent gleam…and Beige Bazazz – a shockingly pretty-pale neutral that murmurs Bazazz ever so gently. Try them. All of them. You'll see then why … Bazazz is. Everything else was.

5/10 each

BAZAZZ AGE COLOURS by MAX FACTOR

Above Despite the psychedelic graphics and the name 'Bazazz age colours' these lipsticks were muted compared with what had gone before.

Left A return to a more natural look chimed well with the coming of the hippies.

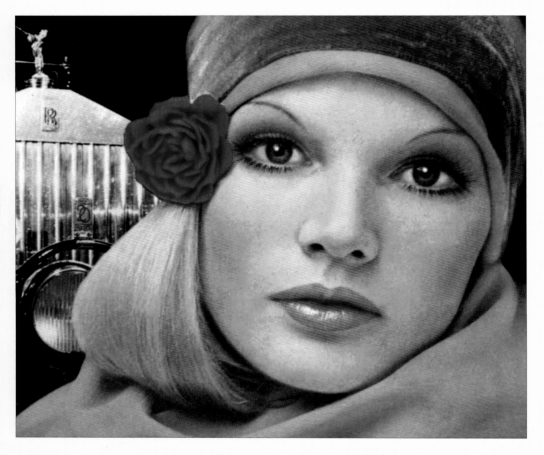

Above *Shiny eyes, shiny lips, shiny skin and pink cheeks – the look of 1968.*

Below *The fashion for shiny skin taken to an extreme.*

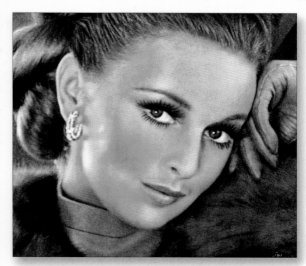

1968 In January **Honey** magazine described the new style: *'Leap into 1968 with a new look, the Moppet look. The face is sheeny, almost shiny; eyes – wide open; cheeks – polished and rosy.'*

'Sling out the heavy black liners; we're concentrating on just making our brush work lighter, buying more muted colours, maybe substituting liquid shadow for liner for an even softer look. New eye-shadow buys will be beigey browns, or clear, sheeny, almost transparent colours. Keep your fake lashes, you're going to need them. Put them on Cathee style or, if you just haven't the time, use loads and loads of lash-lengthening mascara.

'Lips are brighter, it's true, but old-style red lipsticks just don't work. Textures have improved enormously since the last time round. For the pearly-pale colours, the lipstick-makers had to evolve a finer formula, to stop them looking chalky. The '68 "Moppet" has lips that are bright, but with a new, almost transparent glossiness. Salvage old-style red lipsticks though, by putting on, blotting until the "goo" disappears, then polishing off with lip gloss or a pearly slicker.'

Woman's Weekly gave its readers a *'Special tip: Set your foundation by lightly glazing over it with an ice cube. Note: If blusher is used, apply it at this point, and powder over it later.'* That year's **Boyfriend Annual** took up the theme: *'Don't drag the Creme Puff over your face, pat the puff around the face until you have covered the whole surface. Now – the final touch. Sweep over your face with a specially-curved complexion brush to give an unblemished smooth finish to a lovely complexion.'*

'If you use Pan-Cake make-up or Creme Puff make-up, apply cream rouge first. The consistency of cream rouge makes it easy to spread over the skin's clean surface, and then, when the foundation make-up is applied, the result is a natural-looking effect. Dry rouge should be applied after all your make-up – including lipstick – has been entirely completed, and after you have decided what colour clothes you are wearing. Use a thick sable brush and brush on the dry rouge lightly, softly, gently to create the softest glow of colour. Colourful tips: Lightly rouge a prominent lower jaw to call attention away from it. A light blend of rouge at tip of a long nose will make it seem shorter. Newest news in rouge … rouged ear-lobes for a blushing look!'

Woman's Weekly: *'Create a background of colour with eyeshadow. Popular shades of eye-shadow with teenagers are brown and grey for daytime with blues and greens and the iridescent ones for evening or high-spot dates. Stroke the shadow close to the base of the lashes. Then, with the tip of the finger, shade out along the eyelid towards the outer arch of the eyebrow.*

'Apply eyeliner in long, even strokes to prevent flaking or running. If your skin is oily, avoid soft pencil liners – cake types will have more staying power. On the other hand, pencil types tipped with Vaseline or baby oil will help dry-skin eyelids look smooth, soft all day long.' **Boyfriend Annual** added: *'Contour your eyes with eye-pencil, cake or fluid eye-liner applied with a brush. Draw a fine line the length of the upper lid, close to the base of the lashes. Extend the line at the outer end with an upwards tilt.'*

Woman's Weekly gave instructions for applying lipstick: *'Before applying your lipstick, blend a dot of foundation on lips, then dust lightly with powder. This will keep the lipstick from creeping into surrounding pores or wrinkles.'* **Boyfriend Annual** advised: *'Your mouth must not be a gash of colour, but a naturally-tinted feature. Under- rather than over-emphasise. With soft, natural eye make-up, your mouth must balance with a soft, natural lipstick shade. You can use "foundation colours" in both eye make-up and lipstick, provided you don't overdo it. Choose a delicate shade such as one from the three "Young Pretenders" – Beige Pretence, Coral Pretence or Pink Pretence, a youthful range. Apply one coat of lipstick. Blot carefully with a tissue and re-apply.'*

1969 As the hippy style began to take over, make-up either disappeared almost entirely or took on a sultry, romantic tone, often using vivid colours or the smoky hues of the Biba style.

Woman's Weekly recommended a method of making your eyes appear bigger: *'You might try one of the new transparent eye-liners which link with the colour of the eye-shadow you're wearing, so that there's no sudden, hard line. Coty make them in clear blue, clear green, clear grape and bronze, with eye-shadow to match.'*

Woman's Journal in November, gave these tips: *'In spite of all this care taken in applying your eye make-up, it will still run into the surrounding area if previously you have used too greasy an eye-cream, moisturiser or foundation. After you have smoothed in your foundation, blot it very gently with a tissue and hold this tissue underneath your lower lashes while you go through your mascara routine.'*

Woman's Weekly gave advice on improving the appearance of your nails. *'When you apply nail polish, stop just short of each side of the nail. This will give an illusion of narrowness. Let them grow at least an eighth-of-an inch beyond your finger-tips and file them into a pretty oval.'*

Furs were a major part of the romantic look. **Woman's Journal** dismissed the idea that perfume was incompatible with wearing them; *'…perfume may be sprayed on most dark furs, and more delightful conductors of scent are difficult to find. Only the pale furs remain absolutely off limits for fragrance. The way to have a pale fur and perfume too is to scent the lining.'* It also gave a few tips on the subject of economy. *'Put empty scent bottles among your handkerchiefs. Keep your store of scented soaps among your woollens.'*

Left *Rouge, or blusher, was back as cheeks became emphasised.*

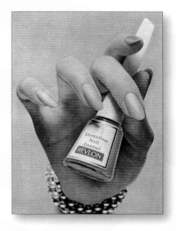

Above *Pearl or frost nail varnish was still fashionable, but like lipstick, natural colours were the most fashionable.*

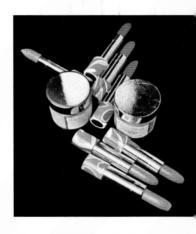

Above *Lipsticks, April 1969, red was back, but smokey purples were the latest colours.*

Conclusion

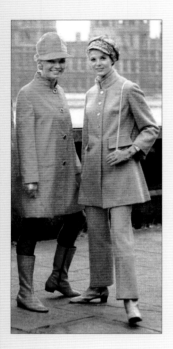

Much like the 1920s, the 1960s are recognised now as a landmark decade, both by those who lived through them and those who came later. Indeed the two decades had much in common; both came on the heels of a world war, both saw huge social upheaval, and both are linked almost inseparably with an adjective – the 'Roaring 1920s' and the 'Swinging 1960s'.

Both saw revolutionary changes led by groups of young designers and artists, the 'bright young things' and the 'beautiful people', who typically rejected the old ways, and embraced a new wave of sexual freedom and experimentation with drugs. Yet in truth neither lasted for a whole decade. The 1960s did not really start to swing until 1963, when the cult of youth took off, and new, young fashion designers blew away the cobwebs and set about smashing all the rules and conventions established by the previous generation.

The search for the new meant that fashions changed at an ever-increasing pace; inevitably this could not last. Designers could not come up with new ideas quickly enough, and genuine innovation gave way to the merely shocking, such as the see-through dress.

The unrestrained commercialism of the new scene also led to a reaction in the form of the hippy movement, whose political radicalism was fuelled by reaction to the Vietnam War and by green issues. Thus the bright sparks of the 'Swinging 1960s' soon burned out, and the final years of the decade took a very different direction.

The 1970s lay ahead, epitomised by mullet hairstyles, platform shoes and unrestrained bad taste. But that, of course, is another story!

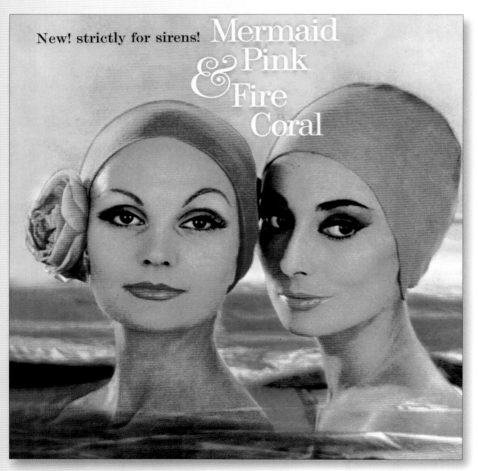

New! strictly for sirens! Mermaid Pink & Fire Coral

The value of £1 in the 1960s

Inflation ran at quite high a rate throughout the 1960s, so year-by-year values are provided here. These figures show (approximately) what £1 then would have been worth today.

1960 – £17.96

1961 – £17.36

1962 – £16.63

1963 – £16.33

1964 – £15.80

1965 – £15.16

1966 – £14.52

1967 – £14.15

1968 – £13.52

1969 – £12.83

Timeline

1960

September – Chubby Checker's version of 'The Twist' reaches No 1 in the USA

November – John F. Kennedy elected president of the United States

9 December– first episode of Coronation Street broadcast on ITV

1961

April – the Bay of Pigs incident, a US-backed attempt to invade Cuba

12 April – Yuri Gagarin is the first man in space

December – the contraceptive pill arrives in Britain

1962

5 October – The Beatles release 'Love Me Do' which reaches No 17 in the charts

5 October – Dr No, the first James Bond film, is released

8–28 October – the Cuban Missile Crisis

1963

12 April – The Beatles release 'From Me To You'. It reaches No 1 on 4 May, where it stays for seven weeks.

7 June – The Rolling Stones release their first single 'Come On' – it reaches No 21 in the charts

June – John Profumo resigns as Secretary of State for War; the 'Profumo scandal' makes a celebrity of Christine Keeler

28 August – Martin Luther King delivers his 'I have a dream' speech in Washington D.C.

October – Harold MacMillan resigns as prime minister due to ill health, and is replaced by Sir Alec Douglas-Home

22 November – John F. Kennedy assassinated in Dallas, Texas

23 November – first episode of Doctor Who is broadcast on the BBC

1964

25 February – Cassius Clay (Muhammad Ali) becomes world heavyweight boxing champion

March, Easter weekend – Mods and Rockers battle in Clacton

May, Whitsun weekend – Mods and Rockers battle in Margate and Brighton

26 June – The Rolling Stones release 'It's All Over Now', which reaches No 1 in the charts

16 October – Harold Wilson becomes the first Labour prime minister since 1951

November – Lyndon Johnson elected president of the United States

1965

March – start of large-scale bombing of North Vietnam by US airforce. US troop numbers in Vietnam increased from 75,000 to 200,000

1966

31 March – Harold Wilson re-elected prime minister

July – football World Cup won by England at Wembley

1967

July – the Sexual Offences Act lifts the ban on gay sex between men. 'The Summer of Love' in San Francisco

October – large anti-war demonstration on the steps of the Pentagon in Washington D.C.

1968

January – start of the Viet Cong's Tet offensive

17 March – anti-Vietnam war demonstration outside the US embassy in Grosvenor Square, London

31 August–1 September – first Isle of Wight rock festival

5 October – major confrontation between civil rights activists and police in Derry, Northern Ireland

November – Richard Nixon elected president of the United States

1969

1–17 August – Woodstock festival, Bethel, New York

12–17 August – political and sectarian rioting in Northern Ireland

December – Provisional IRA formed

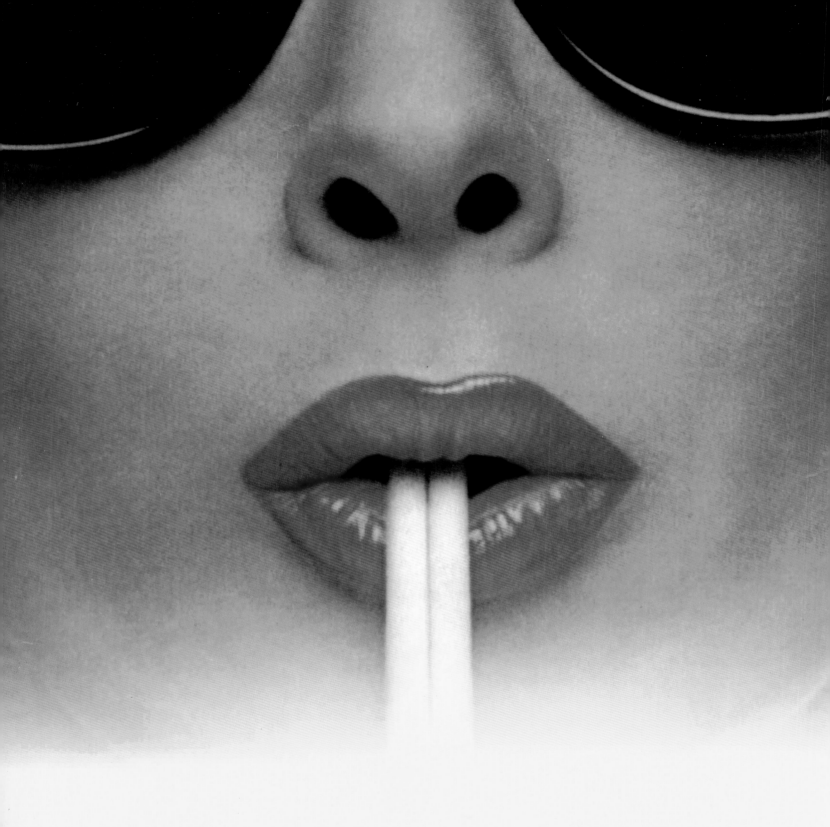

Thanks

I would like to thank the following; the Royal College of Optometrists, Linda Cousins for her photograph on p. 61, Bonnie Walsham for her photograph on p. 111, my publisher Ian Bayley, our designer Philip Clucas, and my family Carol, Will, Raf, and Nadia.